The Arts/Fitness
Quality of Life
Activities Program

The Arts/Fitness *Quality of Life* Activities Program

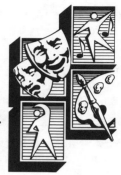

Creative Ideas for Working with Older Adults in Group Settings

by

Claire B. Clements, Ed.D.

Associate Professor and
Quality of Life Program Director
The University Affiliated Program
for Persons with Developmental Disabilities
University of Georgia
Athens

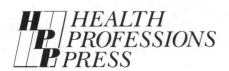
HEALTH
PROFESSIONS
PRESS

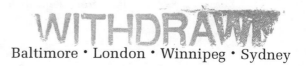

Baltimore • London • Winnipeg • Sydney

Health Professions Press, Inc.
Post Office Box 10624
Baltimore, Maryland 21285-0624

Typeset by Signature Typesetting and Design, Baltimore, Maryland.
Manufactured in the United States of America by
Versa Press, Inc., East Peoria, Illinois.

First printing: January 1994
Second printing: April 1998

Library of Congress Cataloging-in-Publication Data

Clements, Claire B.
The arts/fitness quality of life program : creative ideas for working with
older adults in group settings / by Claire B. Clements.
     p. cm.
  Includes bibliographical references and index
  ISBN 1-878812-14-9 (spiral) : ISBN 1-878812-45-9 (pc)
  1. Aged—Recreation. 2. Physical fitness for the aged. 3. Quality of life.
I. Title
GV184.C54   1994
790.1'926—dc20   93-48044
                                                      CIP

British Library Cataloguing in Publication Data
are available from the British Library.

Contents

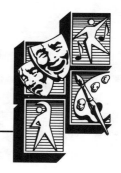

About the Author

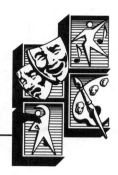

Claire B. Clements, Ed.D., Associate Professor and Quality of Life Program Director, The University Affiliated Program for Persons with Developmental Disabilities, University of Georgia, 850 College Station Road, Athens, Georgia 30610

Claire Clements has been with the University Affiliated Program at the University of Georgia since 1979 and has been the University Affiliated Program Staff Development and Technical Assistance Coordinator since 1986. She has consulted and worked with various programs for 70 federal, national, state, and local agencies. Dr. Clements authored the proposal that resulted in the Project of National Significance grant award from the U.S. Department of Health and Human Services, Administration on Developmental Disabilities that made *The Arts/Fitness Quality of Life Activities Program* possible. She directed the 3-year project and created the Quality of Life manual from the lessons that the Quality of Life staff created and tested at centers and facilities for older adults.

Dr. Clements gives workshop presentations on The Arts/Fitness Quality of Life Activities Program at national conferences. She is a member of the University of Georgia gerontology faculty and was awarded a Georgia State University Gerontology Fellowship sponsored by the National Agency on Aging. Her grant awards in the area of aging include directing the National Endowment for the Arts project, "Art for Older Americans," which served 250 senior citizens in Georgia.

With Diane Barret, Dr. Clements authored "Wellness Express," an interrelated program of fitness and creative arts activities for senior citizens in Georgia. Her Quality of Life team authored "Connecting Commitment II: Five Regional Quality of Life Workshops Across Georgia." She received a grant award from the U.S. Department of Health and Human Services, Administration on Aging, entitled "Quality of Life: A Series of Nationwide Aging and Arts Therapies Video Teleconferences," which will take place in the fall of 1994. Dr. Clements is also the project director for the University Affiliated Program grant award from the Administration on Developmental Disabilities entitled, "Training Initiative on Aging and Developmental Disabilities: Individual-Centered Planning and Supports."

Contributors

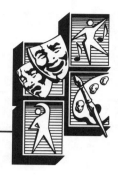

Diane Barret, Ed.D., The University Affiliated Program for Persons with Developmental Disabilities, the University of Georgia, 850 College Station Road, Athens, GA 30610. Barret contributed to the Appendix and to the art activities.

Cal Clements, B.A., 687 Nantahalla Ave., Athens, GA 30601. Clements contributed to general book editing.

Robert Clements, Ph.D., 155 Bar H Court, Athens, GA 30605. Clements contributed to Chapter 3 and to the art and drama activities.

Julia Coleman, M.Ed., 810 Caliber Creek Parkway, Roswell, GA 30076. Coleman contributed to Chapter 3 and to the fitness activities.

Kathy Goff, Ed.D., College of Medicine, The University Affiliated Program of Oklahoma, P.O. Box 26901, BMSB-374, Oklahoma City, OK 73190. Goff contributed to Chapter 1 and to the drama activities.

Sharon Jacobson, M.A., The University Affiliated Program for Persons with Developmental Disabilties, the University of Georgia, 850 College Station Road, Athens, GA 30610. Jacobson contributed to Chapter 3 and to the drama activities.

Michelle McDaniel, B.A., Betty Stockman School of Dance, Calendar Court, Columbia, SC 29206. McDaniel contributed to Chapter 3 and to the dance activities.

E. Paul Torrance, Ph.D., Georgia Studies of Creative Behavior, 183 Cherokee Ave., Athens, GA 30606. Torrance contributed to Chapter 1.

Yunyu Wang, M.F.A., Department of Theatre and Dance, Colorado College, Colorado Springs, Colorado; and Dance Department, National Institute of the Arts, Taiwan, Republic of China. Wang contributed to Chapter 3.

Martha Washington, Ed.D., School of Health and Human Performance, Department of Physical Education and Sports Studies, Physical Education Building, the University of Georgia, Athens, GA 30602-3651. Washington contributed to Chapter 3 and to the fitness activities.

Acknowledgments

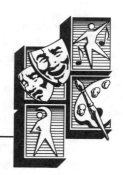

The Quality of Life Program team is made up of people who worked together planning, attending meetings, conducting workshops, teaching lessons, testing subjects, collecting data, and directly or indirectly contributing to this book: Julia Coleman (fitness); Diane Barret, Toni Carlucci, Lara Clayton, Tabitha Carsten, Nina Inman, Corinne Marr, Lilyan Hanberry West, and Sue Ann Nelson (art); Kathy Goff, Margaret Keister, and Jamie McCracken (creativity); June Nail and Valerie Taylor (drama); and Michelle McDaniel, Cynthia Jarvis, Dixie Mills, and Amy Boozer Williams (dance).

The Arts/Fitness Quality of Life Program was implemented with cooperation from individuals in the following agencies: the Georgia Department of Human Resources (Ann Dandridge, Charles Kimber, Chris Robbins, and Bob Herrin); the Northeast Georgia Agency on Aging (Gayle Keeling); and the Athens Community Council on Aging (Kathryn Fowler).

The following senior and service centers participated in the Quality of Life Program: the Greene/Oglethorpe County Service Center (GRO Industries) (Linda Towns Lloyd, Brenda Woods, Shirley Kelly, and Geneva Wright); the Greene County Senior Center (Vivian Murray, Annie Lois Grant, and Clara Wright); the Madison County Service Center (Fine Finish) (Layne Chastain and Mary Jean Booth); the Madison County Senior Center (Eloise McCurly); the Hall County Service Center (Parkway Enterprise) (Michael Byrd and Brenda Beavers); the Hall County Senior Center (Susan Ferrell and Joyce Ann Ray); Guest House (Susan Duffey, Linda Morris, and Beth Sinquefield); the Jackson County Service Center (Solartech) (Mark Stricklett, Susan Morris, and Barbara Reid); the Jackson County Department of Recreation; the Newton County Council on Aging (Josephine Brown); the Dudley Park Senior Center (Marsha Collen and Gayle Sheats); and the Athens Adult Day Care Center (Linda Gough, Meryl Graham, and Carolyn Griffith). Nancy Lett coordinated agency schedules.

Many thanks to all of the senior citizens who have participated in the Quality of Life Program.

The University Affiliated Program for Persons with Developmental Disabilities (UAP) located at the University of Georgia carried out this project in conjunction with the senior centers and service centers cited in these acknowledgments. The UAP has as its major responsibilities the interdisciplinary training of university graduate and undergraduate students, statewide and nationwide dissemination of information, technical assistance, and provision of exemplary service programs for persons with disabilities and their families. The director of the Georgia UAP is Zolinda Stoneman, a nationally known scholar and writer. UAP Exemplary Service Projects include a Training Initiative on Person Centered Futures Planning on Aging and Developmental Disabilities, and the Arts/Fitness Quality of Life Program, Grant No. 90DD0148, funded by the U.S. Department of Health and Human Services, Administration on Developmental Disabilities.

The national clearinghouse for media and print materials related to developmental disabilities, Project STARS, is operated by the UAP and offers the Arts/Fitness Quality of Life Program videotapes. Project STARS can be reached by mail at 850 College Station Road, Athens, Georgia 30610, or by calling (706) 542-6629.

Part I

Using the Arts/Fitness
Quality of Life Program

Introduction

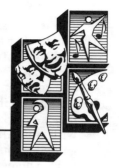

Chapter 1

The *Arts/Fitness Quality of Life Activities Program* is designed to be a practical source book of ideas to assist in developing interdisciplinary programming for older adults. The majority of this manual consists of activity plans in fitness and the arts that were created to strengthen the links between healthy bodies and healthy minds and emotions. These activity plans, presented in Part II, can be viewed as both a springboard of inspirational ideas from which the user and older adults can form exciting activities that are appropriate to their specific needs and as lessons ready to be carried out immediately.

Part II of this manual is organized by months, and each month includes activities in each of four disciplines: fitness, drama, art, and dance. Each activity or lesson is related to the theme or themes noted for the month. These themes help the user to move from discipline to discipline, week by week, and to combine all the disciplines together into final presentations. For service providers, who by the nature of their jobs provide integrated programming, the themes should be most useful.

These themes were designed to tap universal emotions and to appeal to people from all walks of life. This book is specifically designed to facilitate the inclusion of older adults with disabilities, dementia, and losses due to the process of aging. Sometimes special adaptations have to be made to the lessons to accommodate these persons. When this is necessary, suggestions for making adaptations are presented at the end of the activity. For those participants using wheelchairs, three approaches, which vary according to the extent of the participants' limitations, can be followed during activities that involve leg movements.

1. If the exercise involves marching, an individual with some mobility in the lower extremities may participate by alternately raising the heels of the floor or foot rests.

2. Individuals in wheelchairs may engage their upper bodies in as much of the activity as possible. For example, if the group is marching vigorously, participants in wheelchairs can vigorously perform the actions the arms make when marching.

3. Participants in wheelchairs may vary the activity slightly. For example, if the activity calls for marching in a circle, individuals in wheelchairs may move their wheelchairs in a circle to follow the pattern started by those on foot.

The leader should review each activity ahead of time and determine the best way to alter movements so that individuals in wheelchairs may participate fully in the activity.

The presentation and topic of the activity must be concrete. If imaginary and conceptual concepts or concepts relying on memory are included in the lesson, a tangible, current equivalent should be used. All activities should be hands-on. Having a friend help or a leader model the activity will help people with disabilities and dementia. In this way, persons with disabilities can be guided through the activities. It is not expected that people with mental retardation or dementia will acquire what older adults without disabilities or dementia do from the lessons, but they will benefit from the sessions.

Users of this manual should incorporate their own style; the text should not be followed exactly. The book intends to supply new ideas and avenues, not a rigid formula. The lessons contain ideas that were developed in a specific way, but that does not mean it is the best way, the only way, or the way for everybody. Ideas should be adapted to individual styles and methods.

THE ARTS/FITNESS QUALITY OF LIFE ACTIVITIES PROGRAM

The Quality of Life Program is a vehicle for expression and creativity. Participants with and without disabilities derive much pleasure from arts and fitness experiences. Through the ages, fitness, art, drama, and dance, the four creative disciplines in this manual, have been used as a means of communication and expression. Indeed, the arts may be considered the humanities' oldest body of resources for expression and self-realization. Yet, traditionally, creative arts therapies have not been used as techniques with older adults with disabilities. Based on the first implementation of the Quality of Life Program in 1990, it is clear from participant and service provider feedback that participation in interdisciplinary creative arts activities has positive effects.

For maximum benefit, each Quality of Life session must be preceded by a fitness lesson. The fitness lessons utilize themes that foreshadow the next lesson. When fitness is combined with creative therapy, the goals are as follows:

Improved levels of physical, psychological, and social well-being that lead to happier, healthier older adults

Significant changes in life satisfaction, self-concept, and loneliness—as well as achievement of status, prestige, and self-fulfillment for older adults

Improved memory; increased verbal and cognitive skills; improved communication, group skills, and socialization; and the acquisition of emotional outlets for older adults

Achievement of new sources of joy and pleasure; healthier, more meaningful recreation and leisure time for older adults

Increased skills for service providers and leaders in affecting clients' physical, mental, emotional, and social well-being

Increased opportunity in programs to meet varied needs of diverse types of clients

Improved standard of care provided in gerontological settings and increased vision of how to design and implement comprehensive programs

During the Quality of Life Program, democratic procedures should be used for older adults and leaders to jointly choose topics and activities season by season, theme by theme, and lesson by lesson. It is hoped that, together, users of this manual and older adults will gradually expand the areas and activities that successfully tap sources of creative energy and power.

HOW TO USE THIS MANUAL: INTERACTIVE PROGRAMMING

Each month should begin with a presentation to a committee of both older adults with disabilities and those without disabilities of the lesson ideas for that month. Similar to participatory management practiced in Japanese companies, older adults should have a great amount of say in the arts and fitness lessons. When those who use the program invest in the creation and implementation of that program, they get more out of it because the program more directly meets their needs and interests and they participate more readily and in greater depth. With interactive programming and total involvement, the lessons become more meaningful.

Monthly meetings should be scheduled with either the entire group or a committee of adults representing all of the constituents. This is the time to introduce the program and the lesson plans in the book and to listen to the participants and their needs. What do they want to do? Which lesson is their favorite? Would they like to do something similar or based on an activity? As a group, the activities can be adapted so that they address specific individuals in the group, the region and culture in which the group lives, and the concerns of the times. Self-determination and voting are important options to all members of society. By deciding which lesson they want to do, the adults are more invested in the activity. This will whet their appetites. The overall idea is to make the lessons their own; anything that can be done to make the participants feel more invested in the activities should be done. Participants should be encouraged to bring in some of their own belongings as objects to draw in art, as costumes and props in drama, and as music or special dance steps in dance.

Each lesson is designed to integrate older adults into a world bigger than their immediate environment. This manual employs Dr. E. Paul Torrance's incubation model of teaching creativity to meet this end (Torrance & Safter, 1990). The model has three stages: before, during, and after (or beyond) the lesson. The first stage, *before,* inspires the participants and warms them up to the activity. The first stage may take the form of an experience in the community, movement to music that they have brought in, reminiscence about their childhood, or special encounters with the very materials that they will use later in the lesson.

In the second stage, *during,* the participants dig deeper into the subject. They explore different ways of understanding the subject. This is usually the "how-to" of the lesson, or the steps on how actually to do the activity.

The third stage, *after,* is also referred to as "keeping it going" or "beyond the lesson." The information gained in the second stage, *during,* must be given personal meaning. The goal in the third stage is to get the participants excited about finding out more about the subject on their own. This stage should provide the fuel for further investigation. Therefore, the lesson is not over at the end of the activity session, but continues on into their daily lives. Each lesson plan explicitly points out the before, during, and after stages. The incubation model is an important way for the lessons to reach and improve the quality of the lives of older adults.

Another important way to improve the lives of older adults is by use of the fitness program. Along with arts programming, fitness lessons are included in this manual. The lessons incorporate the same monthly themes as the arts lessons and, therefore, fit easily before any other lesson chosen. In order to affect the overall lives of the participants, fitness needs to be performed three times a week or more for a minimum of 20 minutes each time. Because muscle activity gets the blood moving and the body relaxed, an adult's overall creativity, creative flexibility, and creative fluency is significantly improved. Therefore, a fitness lesson should always precede the day's arts lesson.

It is suggested that users of this manual read through each activity thoroughly before presenting it. When necessary, safety precautions are noted at the end of the activity.

BRAINSTORMING AND ASKING PROVOCATIVE QUESTIONS

As noted earlier, the activities in this manual should be adapted to individual styles. This means being creative and capable of problem solving. Brainstorming and asking provocative questions are two ways of generating ideas and solving problems.

Brainstorming

Brainstorming is the unrestrained offering of ideas or suggestions by all members of a conference to seek solutions to problems. Brainstorming is involved in each of the steps of creative problem solving; therefore, it is a basic skill. It can be a warm-up activity or a valuable idea-generating tool.

Brainstorming was introduced by Alex Osborn (1963) as an element of the creative problem-solving method. Brainstorming can be used successfully to stimulate the generation of ideas and facilitate their expression. According to Torrance (1979), brainstorming skills can be developed when practiced with content or when practiced solely for skill development. It is an excellent technique for strengthening imagination, flexibility, and discussion skills.

The heart of creative problem solving is the generation of many alternatives, some of which go beyond the logical and rational. The technique of brainstorming not only improves our ability to *generate* alternatives, but also to *consider* many alternatives. Brainstorming is one of the most teachable procedures for deliberately increasing the number, originality, and quality of alternative ideas.

Four basic rules govern this process; the success of these rules depends upon the degree to which they are applied.

Rule 1. Criticism Is Ruled Out   Do not criticize or evaluate any idea produced; accept any and every idea. This is one of the most important rules and one of the most difficult to master.

Rule 2. Free-Wheeling Is Welcome   The wilder the idea, the better. Off-beat, impractical, silly ideas may trigger a practical breakthrough idea that might not otherwise occur.

Rule 3. Quantity Is Desired   The greater the number of ideas produced, the greater the likelihood of useful, original ideas. This includes bringing out obvious, small ideas as well as wild, unusual, and clever ideas.

Rule 4. Combination and Improvement Are Sought   Combine, "hitch-hike," improve, and change ideas; new ideas lead to more new ideas. Group members are encouraged to "hitchhike" or think of ways in which the ideas of other members can be turned into better ideas, or how two or more ideas can be combined into a still better idea.

It is important to record every contribution on a tape recorder, paper, blackboard, or flip chart. If the flow of ideas slows down or stops, the facilitator may ask questions to stimulate the flow. What if it was much larger or smaller? What if it was a different color or multicolored? What might be some other uses?

The brainstorming technique gives learners the opportunity to use more brains than one. By generating a multitude of ideas, at least one of them will turn out to be useful, innovative, and workable. Asking learners for their input gives them an added sense of importance and creates an atmosphere for creative and imaginative ideas to surface and be acknowledged.

Brainstorming can be used anytime there is a gap in information, a problem, or a question. It is a technique that can be used individually or in groups. Brainstorming provides the opportunities to experience active learning and participation. It stimulates and generates enthusiasm and it promotes spontaneity and creativity. Learners develop an ability to see things from many points of view and to experience a supportive environment for their creative expressions. The Quality of Life study found that creativity scores in fluency and flexibility were increased as a result of the program. Specifically, these scores increased for older adults without developmental disabilities and older adults with developmental disabilities when they were worked with one on one.

Asking Provocative Questions

Almost every facilitator could improve creatively immediately by asking more provocative questions. Doing this makes learning more exciting and increases the acquisition of information, the ability to recall information in problem solving, and the depth of understanding.

Systems for classifying kinds of thinking are useful in generating provocative questions. In a system developed by Benjamin Bloom (1956) and his associates, the major categories are knowledge, comprehension, application, analysis, synthesis, and evaluation. The following can be used as a guide when attempting to think of questions that fall into the last five categories.

1.   Questions requiring depth of *comprehension:*

Translate what is learned from one level of abstraction to another, one symbolic form to another, or one verbal form to another.

Interpret what is learned by explaining, summarizing, or rearranging.

Extrapolate, going beyond the given information, to determine implications, consequences, and effects.

2. Questions requiring *application* of information:

> Go a step beyond translation, interpretation, and extrapolation, showing how information will be used given a situation in which no method of solution is specified.

3. Questions requiring *analysis:*

> Identify and classify the elements involved in a problem.

> Show relationships among the elements and determine their connections and interactions.

> Discover the organizational principles involved, and the arrangement and structure of a body of information or a problem.

4. Questions requiring *synthesis:*

> Recombine previously learned information with new information into unique or original ideas, a plan or proposed set of operations, or a set of abstract relations.

5. Questions requiring *evaluation:*

> Show an awareness of problems, deficiencies, and any gaps in information.

As a result of formal schooling, learners often suppose that any question has a single correct answer. Thus, they need to be encouraged to think divergently. Types of divergent thinking are:

Fluency: Production of as many ideas as possible, quantity not quality is important

Flexibility: Shifting to a variety of approaches or categories

Originality: Unusual or uncommon ideas

Elaboration: Working out the details of an idea

Alex Osborn (1963) recommended the following set of questions to motivate divergent kinds of thinking:

What would happen if we made it larger? Smaller?

What could we add? Take away? Substitute?

What would happen if we took it apart? Rearranged it?

What would happen if we multiplied it? Changed its position?

What would happen if we gave it motion? Odor? Light? Sound? Different color?

What would happen if we changed its shape? Made it stronger? Put it to other uses? Made it of different materials?

After working for a while (e.g., a few days, a week) at asking more provocative questions, progress should be checked. Questions can be written and analyzed according to the different types identified to see what percentage of them fall into each category. Progress can be charted

For practice, provocative questions can be created about simple objects, such as ice, apples, or tin cans. If done as a group activity, group members can analyze one another's questions and get ideas from one another.

REFERENCES

Bloom, B.S. (Ed.). (1956). *Taxonomy of educational objectives. Handbook I: Cognitive Domain.* New York: David McKay.

Osborn, A.F. (1963). *Applied imagination* (3rd ed.). New York: Scribners.

Torrance, E.P. (1979). *The search for satori and creativity.* Buffalo, NY: Creative Education Foundation.

Torrance, E.P., & Safter, H.T. (1990). *The incubation model of teaching: Getting beyond the aha!* Buffalo, NY: Bearly Limited.

Working with Older Adult Learners

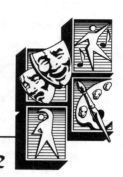

Chapter 2

All adults will be teachers or facilitators of learning at some point in their lives. Some adults have been formally trained as teachers, but most have not been trained, formally or otherwise, as facilitators of learning. To be a facilitator of learning, one must view the learner as a fellow human being in search of knowledge and skills.

A teacher presents certain materials to the learner that he or she determines the learner must know or learn. The teacher takes the responsibility for the learner's learning. The facilitator gives the responsibility for the learning *back to the learner*. The facilitator guides the learner in his or her search for better understanding of knowledge and skills and encourages the learner to seek truths as he or she sees them.

The role of the facilitator is to support the learner as he or she assumes more responsibility for his or her own learning. Eventually the facilitator becomes a resource person for the learner who has discovered how to direct his or her own learning. The facilitator "stretches" the learner to see him or her from different points of view, different angles, and to gain a better understanding of the learner's own perspectives and points of view. Supportive, encouraging, exhilarating, caring, fun, exciting, and life-saving are words that describe a good facilitator of learning.

Some important tips for becoming a good facilitator include:

- Become genuinely interested in other people.

- Smile.

- Remember names—a person's name is to him or her the sweetest and most important sound in any language.

- Be a good listener and encourage others to talk about themselves. Draw from their experiences.

- Talk about the other person's interests.

- Make the other person feel important; do this sincerely.

Also of importance is the ability to change people without giving offense or arousing resentment. Some tips include:

- Begin with praise and honest appreciation.
- Ask questions instead of giving direct orders.
- Be cautious of the other person's ego.
- Praise the slightest improvement and praise every improvement. Be hearty in your commendation and lavish in your praise.
- Give the other person reasons to be proud of himself or herself.
- Make the other person happy about doing the things you suggest.

Probably one of the most important "tips" in working with learners of any age, and probably the strength of the group's leader, is getting to know the people and establishing rapport with them. By remaining "open" to the adults' cues, leaders develop a deeper understanding of the dynamics in each person's life. The leader can use the Quality of Life Program to help build resilience to life's challenges.

When these tips for becoming a good facilitator are used, a major part of the work is accomplished. To complete the task, tips that were learned while doing the lessons with older adults are described on the following pages.

THE ROLE OF PRAISE

Providing encouragement to participants is an important aspect of success as a Quality of Life leader. Thoughtful praise may be the most important factor in making this program work. A study of leadership practices found that athletes whose coaches gave lots of encouragement and positive reinforcement enjoyed the sport and their teammates more than did athletes who received less support (Smith & Smoll, 1984). It is important to find at least one element of the older adult's performance, idea, or product that can be praised. A teacher, when facing a silent class after posing a question, might say, "I really appreciate the time you are taking to think this through. It would have been easy to shout out something without thinking. This shows me you have the ability to concentrate." Even with silence, one can find something to praise.

When learners complete a work of art or project from a lesson, there is a part of themselves in that work. Criticism can be taken by the learners as an indictment against themselves. It does not take much criticism to convince the learners that they do not have good ideas. There may be many faults with their work, but if they receive some acceptance through praise then they do not have to set up their defenses to ward off attack and are more willing to examine their ideas in a meaningful manner.

In searching for the positive, it is important to:

Look at the parts that contribute to the whole.   A participant may show terrific insight even if the end product is not worthy of praise.

Look at the finished product.   Many participants stumble through a creative process, seemingly muddled, yet emerge with a wonderful product. That finished product should be praised first, before its parts are critiqued.

Be specific and refer to an identifiable element. Noticing, for example, the sturdy and strong qualities of a representation of a wheel in a drawing is better than vaguely remarking, "You drew such a nice machine."

Other stages of feedback may follow praise: clarification, criticism, and amplification. In *clarification,* facilitators attempt to have the student clarify various components of the product or idea. The learners are encouraged to express what they may have thought about, but did not present; to explain aspects of their thinking that led to a particular design; or to elaborate upon certain components that offer insight to the learner as well as the facilitator. The questioning is gentle, not accusatory; the purpose is to have as clear an idea as possible of the intent. Once it is clear, it is accepted.

Although this may seem intuitively obvious, the tone of voice used is crucial to success at this stage. It is an information-seeking spur toward understanding the totality of the product. The facilitator wants to understand the student's view, not give any indication of disapproval through his or her tone of voice.

Learners and facilitators who use this approach report that after clarification they rarely need to include the next stage, *criticism,* because the other person often already recognizes the areas that need improvement. Allowing people to identify weaknesses themselves leads to more self-satisfaction.

When it is necessary as part of the learning or growth process, criticism should be gentle and couched in terms that are nonthreatening. Criticism should not be ruled out; it is dishonest to allow learners to feel that what they have done is sufficient if it is not. (Of course, what qualifies as "sufficient" varies with each individual.) In fact, learners often lose confidence in facilitators who accept everything and who never suggest that the learners may be able to perform even better.

During the stage of *amplification,* comments are made to encourage learners to think further about the proposed solution or the product in order to enlarge their horizons. Although there may be a tendency to seek closure and "finish" the product, in this stage of feedback students learn to seek out more information. Amplification does not point to the lack of sufficient accomplishment, but recognizes that there is always more that can be done.

FACILITATING THE PROGRAM

Several suggestions are listed below for making a program a success. As with any method, these techniques require a great deal of enthusiasm. When older adults experience the energy and commitment of their leader, they will be similarly energized.

- Make sure that all participants understand the purpose of the planned activity— why they will be doing the activity, what is expected from them, and how it will benefit them.

- Demonstrate or model the activity. When participants see the skill they are to perform, they will be better able to direct their learning efforts. Demonstrating the procedure leads to faster comprehension of the activity. Modeling the procedure provides a clear picture of what the adults can expect when they are performing the task.

- When planning lessons, think about safety. It helps to know the participants and their strengths and weaknesses. Could the activity endanger the participants? Generally, older adults know when to stop, so respect their limits. Balance and the hazard of falling are a prime concern for older adults. In addition, art materials should be nontoxic. With common sense and care, leaders and participants will realize only better health from these activities. In addition, safety precautions are noted at the end of an activity when necessary. It is important to read these before beginning an activity.

HOLIDAY TOPICS AND FEELINGS OF LOSS

Many of the lessons in this manual focus on holidays and other seasonal events. The emphasis is largely on celebrating these events in a joyous manner. Yet, many older adults experience grief and feelings of loss during holidays. Holidays remind people of loved ones who have died or are far away. They bring up memories of the way things were and can no longer be. Adults who have outlived many people who were close to them are especially likely to have a difficult time with holiday memories.

Acknowledgment and acceptance of these feelings and memories is recommended, rather than denial or repression of them. After allowing members to share real and heart-felt emotions about the season, advise them of ways to cope with grief. For people who are seriously upset, urge them to join a support group that exists for this very purpose. Suggest that group members create new traditions and new ways to celebrate holidays that are otherwise upsetting. Humor is thought to help greatly in easing the pain of loss.

OLDER ADULTS WITH MENTAL RETARDATION

Special attention must be given when communicating with persons with mental retardation. Speak in sentences that clearly and concisely relay the lesson's instructions. It is important for leaders to listen with special care to the person's responses and statements so that they will be able to understand readily what the person is saying. Converse as two adults rather than as an adult speaking with a child, and use normal speech patterns.

A great way to provide extra care and attention for adults with disabilities is the buddy system. Directors of long-term care facilities and senior centers can identify members who are especially understanding and helpful and ask them to volunteer as buddies to adults with developmental disabilities. The buddy system facilitates the inclusion process, sets a tone of helping and caring, and provides a meaningful experience for those people actively participating as well as those who are just observing.

Another way that is strongly suggested to assist older adults with disabilities to become acquainted with adults without disabilities is to organize group lunches. Inviting persons with disabilities to stay for lunch creates a social, relaxed, and enjoyable atmosphere.

ADDITIONAL STAFFING NEEDS

Some of the lessons in the Quality of Life Program may require additional staff. For example, lessons involving complicated movement (dances) and lessons where the entire group must participate reliably for the project to work would be more smoothly facilitated if group members with disabilities or dementia had someone to model the activity constantly. Certain group members with severe disabilities may require extra and continual guidance.

Four main ways to provide extra care are suggested. First, as mentioned above, is the buddy system. Second, volunteers can be asked to aid in specific lessons or with specific individuals. Third, additional staff may be requested to help with the lessons. Fourth, staff who accompany individuals with developmental disabilities may provide additional assistance.

The following are excellent tips for making an older adult center or long-term care facility inclusive that Phillip LePore and Matthew Janicki present in *The Wit To Win* (1990). (An inclusive facility or center is one where all older adults, including those who have been labeled as having mental or physical disabilities, are accepted and included as equal members and are recognized for what they have to offer).

- Set up a staff-sharing relationship between the long-term care facility or senior center and the developmental disabilities center, if possible.
- Inform staff about the participants with developmental disabilities and inform them of any special needs these participants might have.
- Focus on the abilities of the participants while being honest about their limitations.
- Be prepared to be flexible and accommodating.
- Provide individualized training to the people with developmental disabilities in the skills needed for them to make the transition to another environment.

SETTING THE TONE

We hope that the information and ideas provided here will give you the tools to be a great facilitator. As the Quality of Life program has been implemented, it has been found that the person who makes the biggest difference in the success of the program is the director. The older adults see the director as a model and they mirror his or her attitudes. If the director is happy, they are happy. If he or she is open, they are open. However, if the center director is negative or skeptical, they mirror that as well. An exciting and innovative program such as the Quality of Life program requires a general feeling of enthusiasm and openness to succeed. The director/facilitator/leader can create this environment. Here are some final tips to make this happen:

- Talk about what this program can do for the older adults, how much they can get out of it, and how it can improve their overall quality of life.
- Participate in the lessons and ensure that the fitness lessons especially are carried out at least three times a week.
- Provide enough chairs and space for the program to operate.

- Encourage interaction after the activity. Lunch is the perfect time for this.
- Identify the older adults who would be most likely to help this program succeed and give them special coaching on the program. They will then spread good feelings about the program and life in general throughout the center.

REFERENCES

LePore, P., & Janicki, M.P. (1990). *The wit to win: How to integrate older persons with developmental disabilities into community aging programs.* Albany: New York State Office for the Aging.

Smith, R., & Smoll, F. (1984). Leadership research in youth sports. In J.M. Silva & R.S. Weinberg (Eds.), *Psychological foundations of sport* (pp. 371–386). Champaign, IL: Human Kinetics.

Introduction to the Disciplines

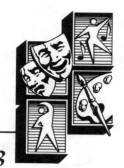

Chapter 3

FITNESS

Aging is often accompanied by problems less common to other age groups, such as loneliness, declining health, reduction in income, and threatened loss of independence. Older adults need involvement in activities that enable them to develop a more positive view of themselves and the world about them. Fitness activities have this potential. Research has shown that participation in group exercise may relieve or reduce levels of depression, improve self-concept, and promote social interaction among individuals within the group. The exercise session should be a period during which individuals can be distracted from daily cares and concerns and fully participate in the joy of movement. The leader has the potential to make these sessions fun and enjoyable while contributing significantly to the participants' quality of life.

GOALS OF FITNESS ACTIVITIES

The quality of life during the older years is influenced significantly by one's ability to remain physically active. Therefore, one of the primary goals of any fitness or exercise program designed for older adults is to provide opportunities that will assist them in maintaining the ability to move efficiently and independently. Participation in an exercise program on a regular basis has been found to promote the maintenance of joint flexibility, muscular strength and endurance, and cardiorespiratory efficiency. Although decrements occur in each of these areas with aging, it is well documented that regular exercise slows or retards the physiological decline.

GENERAL GUIDELINES FOR CONDUCTING FITNESS ACTIVITIES

Several guidelines should be followed when conducting fitness activities:

- Individuals within the groups will be in various states of physical condition. Do not expect all of them to react and perform at the same level.
- Be aware of and sensitive to the fact that the group comprises individuals with varying needs. Be responsive to their individual differences.

- Show respect and appreciation for each member of the group. Too often older adults are treated like children rather than adults.

- Be enthusiastic when leading fitness activities. The group will sense the enthusiasm and want to share it.

- Keep the lessons imaginative to ensure fun, flexibility, and creativity.

- Assume a position in front of the group that allows everyone to see and hear.

- To add variety to the exercises, use scarves, small towels, wooden dowels, or other objects.

- Encourage input from the participants about the types of activities they enjoy.

- Create an environment in which the individuals feel comfortable, supported, and accepted.

- Remember that the purpose of the exercise program for older adults is to move all joints through their full range of movement, to improve muscular strength and endurance, and to promote aerobic capacity (if prior medical screening permits).

MATERIALS AND MUSIC

Special materials required for the fitness lessons are listed at the beginning of each lesson. Every lesson includes music; therefore, a cassette player, record player, or compact disc player will be needed. Music is an essential part of the fitness lesson. It is important that the music be lively (in order to motivate movement) and special to the older adults. If participants have favorite musical recordings, encourage them to bring them for certain lessons. In many lessons, music that is appropriate for the time of the year and the theme of the lesson is suggested. These suggestions are just that—suggestions. Have fun with your music selections. This can be an opportunity to share interests with the participants.

INTRODUCING EXERCISE

The exercise session should be divided into several phases with a logical sequence of progression within each phase. The fitness levels of many older adults is quite low; therefore, participants should start at a low level and progress slowly. The initial sessions should not be too demanding. Exercises can be performed in a sitting, standing, or lying position. Most of the exercises included in the fitness lesson plans are performed in a sitting or standing position to accommodate groups with limited space or a lack of exercise mats. Exercises may be altered or adapted to meet the needs of a particular group. The primary concern should be for the safety and well-being of the participants. During standing exercises, participants should be encouraged to use the backs of chairs for support when necessary and/or stand with their feet shoulder-width apart to provide a broad base of support. Participants should engage in aerobic activities (activities that significantly increase the heart rate, such as jogging, dancing, fast walking) only if they have been medically screened by a physician. An added safety measure might be to keep heart rates below 120 beats per minute.

The exercise sessions usually consist of the following phases:

Warm-Up   Warm-up exercises prepare the body for more demanding exercises and activities. They serve to increase heart rate and circulation slowly, warm the muscles, and gradually increase the range of motion. The warm-up phase helps to reduce the risk of injury due to the fact that warmed muscles are more flexible as well as more efficient. The warm-up phase should last from 5 to 10 minutes.

Flexibility and Muscle Strengthening   Slow, static stretching is recommended for older adults. One should move to a position of stretch gradually and slowly. The stretch should be held 10–20 seconds. This time interval can be increased as the joint becomes more flexible. In positioning for a stretch, the joint should be moved only in its correct and normal range of movement. Flexibility is specific to the muscle being stretched. All major muscle groups in the body should be stretched individually. The progression of muscle groups exercised should be those associated with the neck, shoulders, arms, torso, hips, knees, ankles, and feet.

There is no one specific exercise that is best for strengthening a certain muscle group; as long as muscles contract, strengthening occurs. Light weights, improvised weights, or elastic bands can be used very effectively by older adults for strengthening the muscles. Improvised equipment may include small cans of vegetables, plastic bottles or jugs partially filled with water, or surgical tubing. Weights should be kept light.

Aerobic Activities   Aerobic activity places demands on the cardiorespiratory system and should be included in the program only if participants have been medically cleared for participation. Aerobic activity provides many benefits; however, participation without physician approval could endanger the well-being of the older individual. Aerobic activities include walking, dancing, swimming, and so forth. When aerobic activity is included in the exercise session, heart rates should be checked regularly.

Cool-Down   The cool down, similar to the warm-up, is an important aspect of the exercise session and should never be omitted. It is a gradual tapering of exercise intensity and may consist of walking slowly followed by a gentle stretching of the muscles used during the main phase of the workout.

Assessing Heart Rate

Heart rate assessment is a tool for self-monitoring that may help prevent overexertion. Heart rate during exercise can be a direct indicator of exercise intensity. It is important that each participant learn how to take his or her pulse accurately and with confidence.

Pulse taking is usually accomplished before, during, and after an exercise session to determine the difference between the heart rate at rest, during exercise, and after recovery. There are several places on the body where the pulse can be felt.

To find a pulse, a skill that takes some time, one should relax and be patient. The pads of the fingers, rather than the fingertips, should be used to feel the pulse. Do not apply pressure because too much pressure may reduce blood flow and make it more difficult to feel the pulse.

Where to Find the Pulse   To assess the heart rate at the *wrist,* palpate the older adult's radial artery with your first three fingers. Gently place the fingers

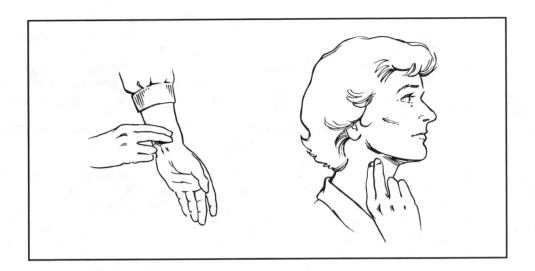

between the tendon and the outside edge of the wrist. Keep the hand and wrist relaxed.

The carotid pulse in the *neck* can be palpated easily, but **be careful** not to depress the artery too much, as this may decrease blood flow to the brain. Depress one side *or* the other, not both.

The heart rate can also be assessed at the *temple* by gently placing the fingers on the temple and feeling the pulse. Again, be careful and do not depress the area too much.

The *base of the heart,* or apex, may also be used to assess the heart rate. Place one or both hands on the right side of the chest under the breast to feel the pulse.

Experiment with palpating the pulse at various sites. Everyone is a little different. Assessing the pulse at the wrist is usually recommended because it is the safest area.

When to Assess the Heart Rate

Rest A resting heart rate is best measured in the morning before getting out of bed. If the heart rate is assessed upon arrival at class, sit down and relax for a few minutes first. A good resting heart rate is 72 beats or less.

Exercise An exercising heart rate should be assessed several times during exercise. The person should keep moving while assessing the exercising pulse rate to prevent going into a recovery heart rate. The exercising pulse rate will vary according to the amount of activity, how accustomed the person is to exercise, and age.

Recovery After completing exercise, a recovery rate should be assessed to see if the pulse is low enough to stop. If the heart rate is greater than 90 beats per minute, it is important to continue cooling down.

How Long to Assess the Heart Rate

All heart rate assessments are based on 60 seconds. The resting heart rate may be counted for 30 seconds and multiplied by 2, or for 10 seconds and multiplied by 6. During exercise, to prevent going into recovery, heart rates are assessed for 10 seconds and multiplied by 6 or 15 seconds and multiplied by 4. The recovery pulse is usually assessed in the same manner as the exercise pulse. Note that the least amount of time for assessments is 10 seconds. (In the past, assessments were made for 6 seconds and multiplied by 10. This made the arithmetic much easier, but the error much greater.)

The following heart rate chart is based on a 10-second count. Multiply by 6 to find the heart rate.

10-second count	Rate/minute		10-second count	Rate/minute
11	66		22	132
12	72		23	138
13	78		24	144
14	84		25	150
15	90		26	156
16	96		27	162
17	10		28	168
18	108		29	174
19	114		30	180
20	120		31	186
21	126		32	192

Note: Participants should have a thorough physical examination prior to beginning an exercise program. In order to participate in aerobic-type activities, a graded exercise stress test is strongly advised.

For people on medication, especially medication that reduces blood pressure, the heart rate chart may offer no parameters for exercise. If this is the case, the individual should work on becoming acquainted with the rate of perceived exertion chart shown below (Hoeger & Hoeger, 1992). The perceived rate of exertion chart provides measures of subjective evaluation of how hard participants are working resulting from subjective association between actual heart rate and perceived exertion.

Rating	Perceived level of exertion		Rating	Perceived level of exertion
6			13	Somewhat hard
7	Very, very light		14	
8			15	Hard
9	Very light		16	
10			17	Very hard
11	Fairly light		18	
12			19	Very, very hard

PROGRESSIVE MUSCLE RELAXATION

The most frequently used procedure for progressive muscle relaxation is an adaptation of the original program described by Dr. Edmund Jacobson (1956). The technique is designed to teach muscle tension awareness and relaxation through alternately tensing and relaxing muscle groups throughout the body. The technique is as follows:

1. Assume a relaxed position lying on the back. Use a pillow if needed. The legs should be straight, arms at the sides, and eyes closed.

2. Practice a few repetitions of the breathing exercises to induce the relaxation response.

3. Remove any distracting thoughts from your mind. Say to yourself, "I am completely relaxed."

4. For each of the following muscle actions, use this procedure: Take a deep breath. Contract the muscles; hold for 5 seconds. Concentrate on the muscular tension developed. After 5 seconds, slowly release the contraction and relax the muscles while exhaling slowly. After exhaling, concentrate on the full state of relaxation in that muscular area of the body.

5. Do the following muscular contractions and movements in sequence, developing the force slowly. Try to isolate the contraction to that body part. Try not to contract other muscle groups.

   a. Curl toes in right foot.

   b. Curl toes in left foot.

   c. Bend right foot upward toward face as far as possible.

   d. Bend left foot upward toward face as far as possible.

   e. Extend right foot downward as far as possible.

   f. Extend left foot downward as far as possible.

   g. Tense upper right leg.

   h. Tense upper left leg.

   i. Tense stomach muscles by flattening lower back against the floor.

   j. Bring shoulders as far forward as possible, keeping head and elbows in place.

   k. Push shoulders back as far as possible, trying to pull shoulder blades together.

   l. Spread fingers on right hand.

   m. Spread fingers on left hand.

   n. Make a fist with right hand.

   o. Make a fist with left hand.

   p. Bring head forward, chin to chest, as far as possible.

   q. Push head back against the mat.

   r. Open mouth as wide as possible.

   s. Pucker lips.

   t. Clench teeth.

   u. Wrinkle forehead.

   v. Close eyes tightly.

DRAMA

There is a distinction between drama and theater. Drama is done for the sake of the participants; theater is done for the sake of the audience. The purpose of a drama activity is in the making, not in the performing. The end product is the experience of the activity. The showing or sharing may come later and be a satisfying way to wrap up the activity, but that is not the drama program's goal. Even if a skit or show is shared later, improvisation and acceptance of new ideas should remain at all stages of the activity. The emphasis should be on being, not on acting. The atmosphere should not change to one that is artificial. There should not be any one person who is the "star"; everyone should take part.

GOALS OF DRAMA ACTIVITIES

The effectiveness of drama to increase the quality of life for older persons is gradually becoming recognized. Participation in a creative dramatics program provides a multitude of benefits. Chief among these is creating an atmosphere of acceptance, comfort, trust, and opportunities for social interaction. Movement and pantomime activities enable the participants to utilize parts of the body that are not often used, and to increase muscle tone, physical agility, and coordination. The therapeutic value of these activities is equally good for people with and without developmental disabilities. For those with disabilities and those who communicate more easily without words, an opportunity is given for expression and communication through the body. Other ways that drama helps the older adult are described on the following pages.

Come to Terms with One's Experiences   Drama helps older adults to gain greater insight into themselves as individuals. It helps them come to terms with their experiences and life situations in a controlled environment. Not only is cognitive loss a problem for many older persons, but so is physical loss due to chronic pain, lack of body awareness, arthritis, visual and hearing impairments, and so forth. Drama helps the older adult become more personally aware of his or her feelings and actions in response to these changes and to gain more awareness of others.

In a sense, drama can be viewed as a rehearsal for life, a way of dealing with the tensions of living together, a way of practicing scripts that run through our heads, and a way of bringing them out into the open for discussion and rational examination. Through drama, one can express one's fantasies, wishes, and fears. It affords an opportunity to express what seems in other situations to be the inexpressible.

Explore Imaginatively   Participating in drama activities is pleasurable. It helps to develop the powers of the imagination. Drama is an extension of play; yet, it is done in a structured, disciplined environment. A simple chair can become a mountaintop or a throne. A sheet or blanket can become the cloak of a notable royal person. A plastic flower could be a wedding bouquet.

Integrate Knowledge and Feeling About Topics   Drama games can help the older adult in his or her efforts to maintain or increase cognitive ability. Reminiscence activities call upon participants to remember things from their past. These memories may be jogged by the feel of something (a scrap of fur to recall favorite pets), the taste of something, or the smell of something (a fresh-baked loaf of bread to recall holiday cooking). Interactions with peers, either a partner or two, can help to reactivate knowledge and feelings about topics. Unlike most other activities, drama is a time to move about, talk, and express emotion. Putting oneself in another person's shoes helps one empathize and understand others. Role-playing increases understanding of a subject, especially when it is followed by a discussion of the issues raised.

Develop Confidence and Ability to Interact in a Social Environment Drama helps participants develop self-expression. Increased self-esteem comes about through having an increased attention span and increased mental alertness. Drama helps adults to overcome shyness. It meets their needs to share and cooperate. Reminiscence and "ice-breaker" activities provide opportunities for social interaction. For many older adults, losses of a spouse, friends, and family are the hardest adjustments to make. Because of the drama program's atmosphere of trust, understanding, comfort, acceptance, and creativity, it facilitates the development of new and meaningful friendships with others.

LEADER'S ROLE

The leader, or activities director, provides and promotes the safety and freedom to do what participants otherwise might feel restrained from doing. The leader's job is to create a mood that encourages sincere effort and establishes trust between the participants and the leader.

A main way to build trust is to have clear goals. It is important to plan a lesson that is not just a disjointed conglomeration of exercises. In stringing together lesson parts to constitute the entire activity, the arrangement of back-to-back activities should not appear random. Instead, in planning the flow of activities from one to the next, devise a scheme that allows participants to see some continuing direction and purpose to the project. Overplan, if necessary. There can always be too much to do, but too little to do can be a disaster. Be prepared; review the activity before starting and have the needed supplies and materials ready and available.

Empower the participants. Allow the participants to suggest lesson ideas; yet, provide guidance in selecting games and improvisations. Ideas can come from the participants, the leaders, and from the manual. Be ready for the unexpected and be prepared to adapt to the situation. Allow the older adults to offer as much feedback and ideas as possible. When the participants feel as if they have ownership in a program, they will be more prone to attend and participate on a regular basis. They will also "market" the program if they believe it is worthwhile. Do not assume the role of artistic director, for the drama program's goal is not to meet the leader's ideas of what is artistic. Instead, raise standards of quality by subtle questioning and discussion.

Always remember to be warm, friendly, and enthusiastic about the activity in order to persuade the participants. If the leader is not having fun, then the participants probably will not either. Be animated and use your whole body and voice to express yourself. Do not destroy the atmosphere of play by a predetermined point of view about the way something should be. Creating an environment where participants feel comfortable and are willing to take risks and to share is difficult. Do not say, "That didn't look good." One way of creating positive attitudes is through consistently validating and reinforcing positive behaviors. Praise, encourage, and reinforce all efforts. Especially encourage evidence of concentration and good group effort.

Dignity

At a time in their lives when dignity is important, older adults are interested in exercises that are sufficiently dignified, not childish. The leader should set up opportunities for participants to gain dignity, not lose dignity. Some exercises can fail when they are below the participants' sense of dignity. Do not ask the participants to do what you would not be comfortable doing.

Specific Teaching Strategies

Some specific teaching strategies are the following:

- Begin the lesson with some casual conversation about clothes, moods, the weather, and so forth.
- Do not be afraid to admit failure and accept responsibility if a proposed activity falls flat. Sometimes even the best laid plans do not work. Say "If this fails, it's my fault; I've picked the wrong exercise. But let's try it anyway and see if it will work."
- Go slowly enough to allow the participants time to create ideas and to act them out before moving on to another phase or idea.
- Let each activity continue until the participants run out of ideas.
- Establish a signal to stop, perhaps a loud clap.

GETTING STARTED

The leader should decide whether it would be easier to get the group to talk or to move first. Music is a good way to facilitate movement. Tell the group to start when the music starts, then as participants get involved in the activity, turn the volume down and let the music be in the background.

Another way to begin an activity is to simulate a morning routine. Lead the group through the many aspects of their morning routine, such as rubbing their eyes, turning on the shower, making coffee, and so forth. Once everyone is "awake," begin the planned activity.

Hand clapping is another way to get the group moving. Try clapping in different positions. Another way to stimulate movement is to make body shapes for each letter of a person's name. Or, try simulating activities that participants have done in their lives, such as hoeing, darning socks, stirring fudge, chopping wood, and shoveling snow. In selecting an activity, try to make it seasonally appropriate.

Mirroring is another way to begin an activity. Ask participants to pair up and have one partner make the mirror image of the movements of the other. Begin with an easy action, such as combing hair, putting on makeup, or shaving. Later on in the lesson, encourage participants to work with a different partner.

Another way to get the group started is to make body movements that express themes such as "the river," "wind," or "fire." Begin by moving one finger to music, then gradually add more fingers, then hands and arms. Keep adding more body parts, while continuing to move those that are already moving. In "The River," for example, first have participants move their fingers for the tributaries, then arms for the river's branches, then their upper bodies for the whole river. Then have them stand up and move their entire bodies. Those participants with mobility challenges should move whatever parts of their bodies they feel comfortable moving. For large movement activities, have participants spread out throughout the room so they will have adequate room to move freely and imaginatively. To minimize self-consciousness, especially at the lesson's beginning, tell participants to turn around so that they cannot see anyone else.

Moving to poetry is another good starting exercise. Be sure to go slowly enough for the participants to come up with their own ideas and to act them out. Alternatively, read a short paragraph from a novel as a starting point. Some participants will be better able to follow just a sentence or a phrase at a time. A short article in the newspaper about a person who did something interesting or unusual can motivate an activity. An article about a social problem that participants are concerned about can be used to trigger role-play; for example, role-playing two bored teenagers about to get into trouble.

PROPS AND VISUAL AIDS

Props and visual aids are useful during drama lessons. For example, pictures of people in paintings can be effective starting exercises. Participants may be asked to dramatize what is happening and what will happen next in the painting. Likewise, cartoons can stimulate the participants' imaginations and can be used for discussions about current situations. Have a selection of sound effects; paintings; quotations from books and articles; music or recorded radio shows; and recordings of natural sounds of birds, animals, the jungle, storms, and ocean waves for use during drama lessons.

Various props can help develop movement and improvisations and motivate participants. Assorted hats, masks, cloaks (from sheets or blankets), belts, crowns, plates, and cups provide the stimulation for movement and role-playing. Any number of items can trigger older adults' imaginations.

A tape recorder is extremely useful in drama lessons. A tape recorder or video recorder is helpful in recording skits for replay and discussion. When recording, observe the counter number when beginning and ending.

DEVELOPMENT AND FLOW OF THE LESSON

The leader describes the activity and offers the stimulation needed to get the activity going. After this, the leader should withdraw and let the participants carry on the activity. It may be necessary to join in occasionally to prod the participants. Knowing when to withdraw and let the group carry the action comes with practice.

In general, individual work is a good way to warm up a drama activity. After a short while, suggest that participants work with partners or in small groups. Differences in group size can be welcome lesson variations and present opportunities for valuable and enjoyable social activity. However, be careful that too many participants working together does not become confusing to the group.

During the second phase of a drama activity, after the warm-up, foster concentration and imagination. Slow-motion exercises are one way to do this. Explore the concepts of time, weight, space, and flow in ways such as the following:

- Practice movements at different heights—close to the floor, medium height, and overhead.

- Practice variations in the speed of the activity—slow-motion, fast-forward speed.

- Practice variations in size and strength, such as that seen in a fire—starting out tiny and flickering, becoming large and strong, fluttering and dying out.

- Practice variations of weight; for example, if the problem was as light as a feather or as heavy as an anchor.

IDEAS AND TOPICS FOR DRAMA LESSONS

Activities can be pantomimed; acted out individually, in pairs, or in trios; acted out in "gibberish" (vocalizations that are not words but that communicate emotions felt); or acted out in a circle with participants facing outward to minimize self-consciousness. Vary the number of participants and the drama modes to keep participants interested. Also, vary the activities by using interesting props. The following list groups a wide variety of ideas for drama activities around six topics.

Fantasy and Imagination

Winning a beauty pageant

What to do about a romantic friend

Landing on an unknown island

What a cat or dog thinks

Winning the million-dollar lottery

An imaginary character going to heaven and meeting St. Peter

Historic Events or Events from Stories

Paul Revere's lookout and ride

Betsy Ross designing the flag

Scarlet O'Hara and Rhett Butler's romance

Personal Insight

A different tomorrow

Why I still have bad habits

Why I am unhappy

Fear of doctors

Conquering a long-standing problem

Social Skills and Activities

Introducing people at a party and telling of their wild, imaginary achievements

Being interviewed on TV for a great accomplishment

Pantomiming a game of checkers or bridge

Meeting people on the street or at the supermarket

Getting a prescription filled or a check cashed

Helping someone to find a contact lens

Striking up a conversation with a stranger

Inviting a friend to a get-together

Asking for, giving, and receiving directions

Visiting a friend in the hospital

Helping a friend close up his or her home and move to another type of living arrangement

Helping a social organization do its work (e.g., helping Habitat for Humanity build a home)

Increasing someone's self-esteem

Accepting praise

Assertiveness

Two people deciding which TV show to watch

Role-playing an owner of a rental house and a disgruntled tenant

Cleaning up the living room together or rearranging furniture

Encounters with social workers and health care professionals

Talking to a Social Security official

Explaining to a banker about a financial matter

Reminiscence

Dialogue and action in the kitchen before a big holiday dinner

Harvesting the crops

Decorating one's living quarters for the holidays

CONCLUDING A DRAMA LESSON

At the end of a drama activity, sum up what happened in the lesson and encourage participants to integrate the material into their lives. Encourage sharing thoughts that the activity brought to mind. Discussions may turn to the wisdom and moral implications of certain story lines. Close the lesson by telling participants to think about how this activity could be part of their daily lives. Or, end the lesson by asking participants to think about what they would like to do that evening or what they would like to dream about that night. Tell them to think about having no worries, taking a hot bath, or looking out at a beautiful view. The drama lesson might blend into a follow-up activity in arts and crafts, poetry, or storytelling.

ART

Opportunities should be available for the creative expression of older adults with and without disabilities at senior centers, long-term care facilities, and adult day-care facilities. In the final stage of life, avenues for fulfillment and satisfaction are needed. Research shows that older adults who participate in art programs live longer than those who do not participate. Therefore, in addition to improving the adult's quality of life, art contributes to longevity. Nine years after an art class was given to a group of older adults, 67% of the participants who had studied oil painting and continued to study were living, as compared to 38% of a control group who had studied no art. Additionally, 65% of the experimental participants were given ratings of "excellent" or "good" on an evaluation of their health, in comparison to 12% of the control group (Dawson & Baller, 1972).

GOALS OF ART ACTIVITIES

Art activities provide many benefits. The purposes of the activities are:

- To exercise creativity, individuality, and imagination
- To exercise perception, cognition, memory, and psychomotor coordination
- To experience feelings of self-expression and emotional support within a caring community by participating in the art activity and sharing feelings about the activity and its recalled experiences with others
- To make an immediate contribution to the environment by individualizing it and beautifying it with creative products
- To carry out activities that older adults feel are age-appropriate, interest-appropriate, and ability-appropriate

LIMITATIONS OF COST AND RANGE OF MATERIALS

Many senior centers, adult day-care centers, and long-term care facilities focus their efforts on nutrition and health programming, and as a result often have little money left for art supplies. Busy staffs operating with limited budgets and limited time to spend acquiring special materials cannot order elaborate art supplies. Therefore, for an art program to be effective in such places, it must require only a minimum of supplies: scissors, construction paper, marking pens, Craypas, glue, and poster paint. Art activities can be more sophisticated if more sophisticated and unusual art materials are available. The adults participating in the activities would probably find elaborate materials more interesting and challenging. Although expensive art materials are exciting to use and result in sophisticated-looking art products, art programs must be designed that can be implemented with low-cost and common materials. The materials need not limit the expressive potential of older artists; folk artists transform unlikely and commonplace materials into objects of profound beauty.

ART FOR OLDER ADULTS WITH AND WITHOUT DISABILITIES

Persons with developmental disabilities should lead their lives in an inclusive environment—one that allows them to participate with people without disabilities. An inclusive environment gives people both with and without disabilities an opportunity to learn from one another and enjoy one another. For those adults who have recently become disabled, seeing how persons with developmental disabilities deal with their disabilities teaches a lesson in fortitude and coping.

To create a program that is appropriate for both populations is a difficult goal to achieve. One route is to have art lessons cut across ability levels by using topics that all persons have experienced throughout their lives. Monthly and seasonally recurring themes are examples of such universal topics. Another approach is to focus the art projects on emotional experiences common to everyone. Despite the best efforts to design lessons to meet the needs of all persons, there may be aspects of the project that are not suitable for some of the group members. Getting started on an art activity is the hardest part for most older adults because they must overcome fears of inadequacy. Just getting the participants to start is often a major goal—one that falls far short of spontaneous self-expression (Crosson, 1976). A fairly high degree of structure and simplicity in the project's beginning alleviates this problem. Persons of nearly all ability levels will be able to undertake a project that they clearly understand and believe they can accomplish. Research on caution in adulthood has shown that older adults, compared to college-age adults, select tasks that present higher probabilities of success (Okun & DiVesta, 1976). Thus, older adults with and without disabilities tend to prefer tasks without a high degree of challenge. Projects presented as fun and uncomplicated motivate both populations to participate, leaving each artist the freedom to develop the project into something as complex and challenging as he or she would like.

Another method of creating art projects for an inclusive group is to include a crafts approach and a painting approach. Some writers advocate a crafts approach because more people, and people with a greater range of abilities, can participate. That is, many older adults will refuse to draw and paint. However, some other adults may not be satisfied with craft activities, which may not integrate the mind and spirit in the same way that painting, sculpture, and other fine arts do.

The art activities in this manual have been designed so that they can be performed by participants with developmental disabilities and include a crafts orientation. Calling for life review and emotional sharing (described in subsequent sections) to manifest itself in crafts projects allows adults to experience the mentally integrating power of fine art.

In some art programs there is a converse and concomitant problem of an insufficient degree of challenge. "Our society badly underestimates the creative and intellectual abilities and desires of the elderly population, with some programs offering little long term intellectual benefit, and only providing momentary diversion. . ." (Hoffman, 1975, p. 21). This manual attempts to resolve this issue in two ways—first, through art, and second, through life review and emotional sharing.

In the sphere of art, a central focus upon imaginatively used art elements, such as shapes, colors, lines, and textures, will allow persons of varied abilities to participate, each at his or her own level. As the activity progresses, the activities director can call for more use of individual imagination with statements such as, "How else can you show this idea using different textures and lines?" "How can you make the composition more dynamic?" Art ideas should be brought out. Participants should be encouraged to extend themselves in their thinking and encouraged to think of repeating elements to create rhythms and interesting designs (Jones, 1980a). Teaching art ideas to older adults is important because they need to have a strong feeling that they are learning, not merely passing the time.

The second way to address the potential lack of challenge in art activities is by having the activity serve as a vehicle for two other important tasks—life review and emotional sharing. Setting aside one's degree of ability, all people experience and have experienced at some time a common ground of emotional responses. Virtually all older adults have the need for reminiscence and life review (Kaminsky, 1984). Creating an art object serves as a facilitating agent, a medium through which these two goals can take form. "Art brings out feelings that need to be expressed and shared, stirs emotions and often evokes fond memories from the past" (Parris, 1986, p. 44). A participant's thoughts and feelings are focused by the creation of a physical and aesthetic object. Thus, whether or not one is challenged by the specific, tangible art construction activity, most everyone can find satisfaction and meaning in emotional sharing and life review.

Life Review

Reminiscence is sometimes thought of as a defect, similar to regression. It is sometimes looked upon with amused disdain and considered to be tiresome self-indulgence and a useless preoccupation with past things, people, and events better left forgotten. However, modern research shows that psychological flexibility, resourcefulness, and optimism characterize older adults who reminisce (Kaminsky, 1984; Moody, 1984).

Researchers present two seemingly conflicting explanations of how reminiscence produces such beneficial qualities. One theory is that by focusing on a happy past, the elderly individual may be tuning out a present unsatisfactory life situation. Bibring's (1961) theory, for example, is that reminiscence helps people maintain their sense of self-esteem by satisfying three desires: 1) to be appreciated or loved, 2) to be strong or superior, and 3) to be good and loving. Older adults look back to earlier times when they were loved, strong, and loving, and bring these good memories into the present. In the present, the memories are further reinforced by their incorporation in tangible art mediums.

Reminiscence plays a central role in Erikson's eighth stage of psychosocial development—ego-integrity versus despair (Erikson, 1982). Ego integrity is the acceptance of one's only life cycle and acknowledgment of one's approaching death. Reminiscence in old age fosters successful adaptation by upholding life-long practices and beliefs, confirming the rightness of one's lifestyle, and conveying a sense of world order and spiritual sense. It reestablishes a comradeship with the ordering ways of distant times and different pursuits, as expressed by the simple products and sayings of such times and pursuits.

Butler (1963) asserts that by reminiscing an older adult works through unresolved conflicts: regret, grief, guilt, and unfulfilled ambitions. For example, Butler states that reminiscence is "characterized by the progressive return to consciousness of past experiences and particularly the resurgence of unresolved conflicts which can be looked at again and reintegrated. If the reintegration is successful, it can give new significance and meaning to one's life, and prepare one for death, mitigating fear, and anxiety" (p. 71). Through art lessons that result in an individual remembering unpleasant experiences, he or she is helped to work through the lingering unpleasant emotions. An unresolved negative event is never forgotten because people tend to mull the event over in their minds, thinking about what they could have said and done. When the event has been given tangible form in art, the individual can attain symbolic mastery over it, see the trauma with a clearer perspective due to greater emotional distance, and break the endless cycle of negative thoughts and feelings. Thus, reflection on unhappy memories in collaboration with art improves mental well-being.

Whether or not reminiscence makes older adults psychologically satisfied through the re-creation of happy thoughts or the redressing of unhappy thoughts or both, it definitely improves their state of mind. Nondepressed seniors tend to reminisce more than those who are depressed. In analyzing the statements of older adults, researchers found that 66% of the statements by people classified as "good copers" related to the distant past, 32% related to the present, and 2% related to the future (Kaminsky, 1984). In other words, reminiscing is an effective way of maintaining good mental health.

In fact, reminiscence is not only an effective vehicle for coping and maintaining mental health, but also for extending life. In the 1-year follow-up study of survival rates, 3 of the 4 older adults participating in the study who had been rated as depressed had died, 4 of the 5 rated as suspected of depression had died, and only 1 of the 16 rated as not depressed had died (Kaminsky, 1984). Because reminiscing alleviates depression, reminiscing seems to extend life.

Alfred Adler (1958) believed reminiscence had a special usefulness. It was not just a helpful tool for life coping, but, for people for whom involuntarily emerging was the key to the very essence of their personality, it was a substitute for their self.

Most of the art lessons in this manual have a component of reminiscence and calling forth from one's life experience some aspect to review and share with the group. By creating some object, drawing, or representation that serves as a tangible vehicle for remembering and discussing one's life, older adults will experience a feeling of satisfaction. Their reminiscences do not need to conform to someone else's standards of accuracy. Additionally, the art object need not portray the memory in specific realistic terms because often even the most powerful memories can be very vague.

> From among myriads of impressions we might remember, there are only a few which actually emerge involuntarily, without any conscious deliberate effort: a shape, a color, a sound, the peculiarly unique quality of a shape, color, or sound, the shred of an occurrence ever so much more insignificant (by official standards) than many events forever forgotten. . . vivid and so gruesomely personal, these memories are one's own self, fair samplings of ourselves, representatives of ourselves as we have unconsciously decided to appoint them as our representatives. (Adler, 1958, p. 9)

Adler believed that involuntary memories, filled with seemingly irrelevant detail, were not only central to a person's identity, but that they could be used, no matter how old the person, as a means of education and clarification of the meaning of life. Therefore, for art motivations the topic should not be narrow and specific, such as "The Ice Storm of 1930." Instead, broad topics, such as "Early Winters I Can Remember," are more effective expressions of powerful, yet vague, memories.

Sometimes an older adult's creativity is manifested beautifully in artistic representations of reminiscences. Many older adults can create beautiful art from memories (Osgood, 1985; Suhart, Campbell, & Vesely, 1977). However, there are many older adults who feel that folk-type representations do not meet their own criteria for proper representation of the human body, and their criticism prevents them from even trying to represent figures in reminiscence themes. They will not draw and will not participate in the activity. It has been pointed out that reminiscing assignments are more threatening than others and more difficult to use (Dewdney, 1973; Jones, 1980b). This is probably because of their fears of showing their lack of ability in art. Perhaps it is also because of psychological conflicts and mixed feelings toward the persons they are to represent. To have the advantages of reminiscence without the disadvantage of lack of participation, it may be best to focus in the beginning of the lesson on the construction of a craft that can be adorned later with drawings, words, and images from one's past.

Emotional Sharing

Older adults should always be encouraged to share their emotions as they participate in art. Emotions connected with the topics should be elicited so that participants can holistically experience therapeutic benefits through a greater sense of integration of their life experiences (Osgood, 1987). Researchers have shown that those who talk with others about the loss of their loved ones are healthier than those who remain silent (Ornstein & Sobel, 1989). Feelings of anxiety, loneliness, uselessness, unwantedness, and guilt, perhaps triggered by family interactions with their grown children (Kodel, 1986), or feelings of disengagement that may mask apathy or rage brought on by social exclusion might be expressed and dealt with in a positive way (Kaminsky, 1984). If themes of loss and death arise, they should be allowed to develop so that group members may provide each other with support (Van der Kolk, 1983).

Talking about problems may be helpful in alleviating depression. One study found more avoidance behavior was used by depressed persons than by nondepressed persons (Foster & Gallagher, 1986). An outstanding example of the harmful effect of avoidance that was overcome through art expression is the case of an older woman with depression who barely talked and had to be hospitalized for schizophrenia for 40 years. Art therapy helped her to express the trauma of a broken heart and subsequently to live outside the institution in a community group home. She spoke most often when she was drawing (Lowe, 1984). Another example of art's power to overcome depression is the controlled experiment that showed that art activity inhibited the development of depression in withdrawn nursing home residents (Wilson, 1983).

The physical decline of an older person often leads to a decreased capacity for relationships both with people and with objects; the subsequent systematic self-restriction only serves to heighten a person's tendency to feel abandoned and alone (Van der Kolk, 1983). These feelings can be redressed while working together creating art in groups, which can give these adults a sense of continuity and usefulness to others. To facilitate sharing, the participants can work together on a group project or with one other person on a joint art activity (Nadeau, 1984). The value of social relationships brought about through art sharing has been recognized by participants who say the classes brought a close relationship and understanding of other people's needs, hopes, and desires. Art helped them to see their common hopes for a better future for all people (Pierce & Burgio, 1981).

Art sharing, which strengthens the individual's social support system, shows how a person can both help another person and turn to another person for help. Thus the individual's self-confidence and coping behavior is strengthened (Clark, 1982). All art lesson plans should include time to share and talk together while warming up to do the project and after the project is complete. Yet, often older adults are reluctant to express the emotions they feel. One way of solving this problem is by interpreting another person's art. Although on the surface it may appear that they are talking about the other person's art, they are also sharing their own emotions. Thus, by talking about some else's art, older adults can safely give expression to their own feelings.

Body Movement

Exercise, affirmations, and guided imagery integrated with art activities can have the potential for improving older adults' well-being (Fling, 1982). Art activities for adults should have some body movement incorporated into them. Movement is done not only for needed exercise, but also to enhance clarity in thinking about the upcoming aesthetic experience. Thus, movement has kinesthetic benefits that get the body and mind "working" at a higher level, and intensify the participants' desire to do the project. Art teachers have seen how warm-up exercises increase the quality of participants' art. As the ancient Greeks believed in "a sound mind in a sound body," art teachers believe that exercise and motion of the body are among the best ways to promote healthy emotions.

Sharing Art

Maintenance of self-esteem is mandatory during the final stage of development. In addition, society must renounce ageist attitudes of decline and uselessness, and provide appropriate opportunities for people who are older to reach out and contribute (Snowdon & Brodaty, 1986). E. Paul Torrance, the noted expert on creativity, has emphasized the need to extend what is done during the lesson to one's ongoing life and the lives of others (Torrance, 1989; Torrance & Safter, 1990). Exhibiting the art of older adults is one way of sharing art with the world. Childhood scenes by folk artists such as Grandma Moses and Mattie Lou O'Kelley are considered national treasures and many generations have benefited from their willingness to share their lives through art.

We can reestablish in a small way how older people functioned in primitive societies as storytellers and carriers of ancestral and tribal lore by making public their art. Ortega Y Gassett's concept of generations is that the same historical events occur to members of a given generation at the same stage of their lives: early adult, mid-life, and so on. These decisive historical events lend each generation its distinct biography, its collective historical character. There is a discontinuity, an incommensurability between generations, that helps to explain why each generation always misunderstands its successor. To see a single generation's task is at the same time to apprehend an entire historical world. This generation, this historical consciousness, is a precious part of the public world (Moody, 1984).

By reproducing the artwork of older persons, art that contains their values, experiences, and ideas, society gains insight into its history and its future. Society must bring together the recollections and writings of older adults, perhaps including them with their art or publishing them in a local paper or newsletter. Art displays can be exhibited at senior centers or displayed to the public in a local library, gallery, theater, restaurant, or school.

Another way older people can feel useful is by actually giving the art products they create to others. Older adults who can give and receive have better self-esteem and function better than those adults who can neither give nor receive (Stein, Linn, & Stein, 1982).

Thus, there are many ways to help older adults share their art and experiences with society. This process improves the quality of life for older adults, who throughout their younger years contributed to the world and need to continue doing so.

DANCE

The dance lessons in this manual were designed for participants to explore movement that involves the emotional, spiritual, and social self. The lessons were built around monthly themes so that the dance lessons could be mixed easily with fitness, art, or drama lessons. They also support one another in a consecutive fashion; therefore, it is beneficial to spend time exploring dance movement during more than one time period.

Many lessons involve the use of imagination. When working with people with disabilities, limit the images; however, do not simplify too much or the challenge will be lost.

Everyone benefits from heightened awareness of basic movement. Movement comes from breath; life begins with breath and ends with breath. Participants should enjoy the experience of becoming aware of their breath and how it changes as well as their own unique movement. Breath consciousness should be a major goal of the dance lessons to assist older adults to gain a sense of self—body, mind, and soul.

GOALS OF DANCE ACTIVITIES

Dance activities are therapeutic, emotionally as well as physically. The purposes of the activities are to improve:

- Fitness
- Memory, coordination, verbal, and cognitive skills
- Communication and social skills
- Self-discovery and expression in dance
- Self-esteem and fulfillment

In general, each activity contains three stages: the warm-up, the main activity, and the cool-down.

DEVELOPMENT AND FLOW OF THE LESSON

Warm-Up

The opening section of the class is used to warm the major muscle groups and allow the participants to "come together" in preparation of the events to follow. The exercises, while allowing capabilities to increase, will remain fairly constant from month to month so that the warm-up will become familiar and almost ritualistic. The familiarity of the routine is comforting to older adults.

The warm-up is designed to focus concentration, bring the body and mind together, capture attention, create a desire to know, heighten awareness and anticipation, tickle the imagination, and warm the body gradually for work in the main activity. Good posture and alignment should be emphasized.

The following exercises can be done sitting, standing, or wheeling, preferably with calm, soothing music. If the adults choose their own music for the activity, they will be more motivated to participate. During the lesson, imagery can be added (e.g., "tilt your head from side to side like a pendulum clock") to increase interest.

1. *Breathing* Take a deep breath and feel the slight lifting of your whole body, then let the air out slowly with the feeling of the torso relaxing. Try the breathing exercise later with the sound of "shhh, ha ha" when breathing out. Count during the exercise and try to increase the time used to inhale and exhale.

2. *Face warm-up* Work the face as if chewing, smiling, kissing, squeezing, and twisting. Move your eyes from side to side, up, down, and in circles. Open the eyes as widely as possible and then close them tightly. Use the eyes to express a variety of emotions, such as anger, sadness, happiness, and frustration.

3. *Neck warm-up* Tilt the head from side to side. Move the head as if to say, "yes," or "no," and circle it from right to left, and then from left to right. Make sure to do the above movements gently and slowly to avoid injury.

4. *Hands* Stretch the hands wide open and then let them go limp. Shake the hands and then roll the wrists in a circular path, right and left.

5. *Shoulder roll and lift* Roll the shoulders forward and then backward. Try moving the left shoulder forward while moving the right shoulder backward and vice versa. Try to shimmy.

6. *Arm and elbow "dances"* Using tension, relaxation, shaking, squeezing, and punching movements, move the arms at will. Reach the arms in different directions. Upper torso movements can be incorporated later.

7. *Knees* Lift one knee up and put it down using different counts to the music, such as a 4, 3, 2, 1 count. Switch knees.

8. *Feet and ankles* Flex and point the foot slowly through each part of the foot: the toes, heel, and ankle. Circle the ankle with the foot to the right and left, then up and down. Squeeze the toes together and spread the toes out.

9. *Torso* In a sitting position, slowly lead with the top of the head to round the torso forward, dropping the shoulder and upper chest to reach down the arms as if picking up something from the floor. Let the torso go as low

as it can without straining. Then reverse this movement, making sure that the head is the last to go upright.

10. *Walking, marching, and clapping to music*   As the classes progress, head and arm movements can be added to walking and marching for more challenge and expression.

Main Activity

The main activity stimulates the imagination; explores body mobility; improves fitness; improves freedom of expression; and creates awareness of force, time, and space. Self-esteem is gained through the no-fail nature of the activities. At the end of the main activity, the participants have a feeling of completion and self-discovery.

This portion of the class will be used to explore a number of different types of movement. Some of the activities that will be experienced include the following:

Storytelling   During story telling, the teacher tells a story while the older adults move individually and according to the story. This stimulates creativity and improves coordination.

Touch Dances   During touch dances, participants move around the room aimlessly and then find a partner and touch them when the teacher cues. This could begin with handshakes; progress to touching elbows, heads, feet, and knees; and then move to hugging. This should be a fun and socially pleasing activity as well as one that allows the body to move freely. Touch dances lend themselves to other activities involving leaning, pushing, and pulling.

Folk Dances and Social Dances   Folk dances and social dances are other group activities that improve mobility and coordination. Special wheelchair dances can be fun to invent and implement. Folk and social dancing provide the opportunity to learn the history related to the dance.

Modern Dances and Ballet   Modern dance and ballet allow the participants to learn and appreciate some basic principles used commonly by professional dancers. They also allow older adults to feel as though they have "learned to dance."

Holiday Dances   Special movements based on upcoming holidays get the participants into the holiday spirit and create excitement and anticipation.

Improvisation   Many of the dance activities already mentioned have improvisational qualities that will serve as an introduction to improvisation. Improvisational activities can be inspired by personal experiences, props, music, graphic designs, or holidays. Improvisation frees the mind and allows the use of the body for self-expression. It encourages creativity, unity, expression, and personal and social satisfaction. Certain movements inspired by improvisation can be arranged into a nonimprovisational dance by the adults.

Cool-Down

The same cool-down technique, mirroring, is used in every session, with slight variations each time. Mirroring is performed with partners at first, then trios, and eventually the entire circle works together mirroring each other's movements. This exercise establishes a strong sense of community. It should be viewed as a social activity.

This is the last part of the class session. It should be simple and slow, and it should allow the dancers to prepare to end the lesson and to leave.

Slow, Easy Stretches Stretching the warm body is the most effective way to increase flexibility. Effective cool-down stretches include lying down; stretching the fingers toward the toes in two directions; or reaching into the air, out to a partner, to the side, or elsewhere.

Mirroring Participants pair up and experience leading, following, and perhaps even simultaneous mirrored movement. The leader pretends to look into a mirror and creates movements. Everyone else—or, if the dancers are in pairs, the other person—mimics the leader's movements as precisely as possible. Concentration, coordination, control, and range of movement should increase. Mirroring, by allowing the students to experience shared movement, increases social satisfaction.

Tai-Chi Concentration and Meditation Tai-Chi is an effortless and rhythmical art that focuses on slow breathing, balanced and relaxed posture, and absolute calmness of mind. The slow, concentrated movements and meditation allow the body to cool down, which can serve as a nice transition from dance class to the next activity.

REFERENCES

Adler, A. (1958). *The education of the individual.* New York: Philosophical Library.

Beck, A. (1975, April). NCAEE…The past is a good beginning. *School Arts,* 42–43.

Butler, R.N. (1963). The life review: An interpretation of reminiscence in the aged. *Psychiatry, 26,* 65–76.

Clark, A.W. (1982). Personal and social resources as correlates of coping behaviour among the aged. *Psychological Reports, 51*(2), 577–578.

Crosson, C. (1976). Art therapy with geriatric patients: Problems of spontaneity. *American Journal of Art Therapy, 15,* 51–56.

Dawson, A.M., & Baller, W.R. (1972). Relationship between creative activity and the health of elderly persons. *The Journal of Psychology, 82,* 49–58.

Dewdney, I. (1973). An art therapy program for geriatric patients. *American Journal of Art Therapy, 12*(4), 249–254.

Erickson, E.H. (1982). *Identity and life cycle.* New York: Norton.

Fling, S. (1982, April). *Creative health for elders through psychology and art: A pilot study.* Paper presented at theSouthwestern Psychological Association. (ERIC Document Reproduction Services No. 234 326)

Foster, J.M., & Gallagher, D. (1986). An exploratory study comparing depressed and nondepressed elders' coping strategies. *Journal of Gerontology, 41*(1), 91–93.

Hoffman, D.H. (1975). A society of elders: Opportunities for expansion in art education. *Art Education, 28,* 20–22.

Jacobson, E. (1956). *Progressive relaxation.* Chicago: The University of Chicago Press.

Jones, J.E. (1980a). The elderly art student: Research and the participants speak. *Art Education, 33*(7), 16–19.

Jones, J.E. (1980b). On teaching art to the elderly: Research and practice. *Educational Gerontology, 5*(1), 17–31.

Kaminsky, M. (1984). The uses of reminiscence: A discussion of the formative literature. *Journal of Gerontological Social Work, 7*(1–2), 137–156.

Kodel, R. (1986). Disturbances in the family situation from the view of the aging person. *Zeitschrift-fur-Alternforschung, 41*(5), 297–299.

Lowe, M.E. (1984). Smoke gets in your eyes sometimes. *The Arts in Psychotherapy, 11,* 267–277.

Moody, H.R. (1984). Reminiscence and the recovery of the public world. *Journal of Gerontological Social Work, 7*(1–2), 157–166.

Nadeau, R. (1984). Using the visual arts to expand personal creativity. In B. Warren (Ed.), *Using the creative arts in therapy* (pp. 61–80). Cambridge, MA: Brookline Books.

Okun, M.A., & DiVesta, F.J. (1976). Cautiousness in adulthood as a function of age and instructions. *Journal of Gerontology, 31*(5), 571–576.

Ornstein, R., & Sobel, D. (1989). *Healthy pleasures.* Reading, MA: Addison-Wesley.

Osgood, N.J. (1985). *Seniors on stage: The impact of applied theatre techniques on the elderly.* New York: Preager.

Osgood, N.J. (1987, June). *Wellness through creative expression in late life.* Paper presented at the ICHPER chapter, University of British Columbia.

Parris, D. (1986). Stimulating creativity through artistic inspiration. *Journal of Gerontological Nursing, 12*(5), 44.

Pierce, N., & Burgio, M. (1981). *Evaluation of the liberal arts program of the international study of older adults.* (ERIC Document Reproduction Service No. 210 056)

Snowdon, J., & Brodaty, H. (1986). The life cycle VIII: Old age. *Australian and New Zealand Journal of Family Therapy, 7*(2), 103–107.

Stein, S., Linn, M.W., & Stein, E.M. (1982). The relationship of self-help networks to physical and psychosocial functioning. *Journal of the American Geriatric Society, 30*(12), 764–768.

Suhart, D., Campbell, M., & Vesely, A.J. (Producers). (1977). *Art in action* [Film]. Athens: University of Georgia Center for Continuing Education.

Torrance, E.P., Clements, C., & Goff, K. (1989). Mind-body learning among the elderly: Arts, fitness, and incubation. *Educational Forum, 54*(1), 123–133.

Torrance, E.P., & Safter, H.T. (1990). *The incubation model of teaching: Getting beyond the aha!* Buffalo, NY: Bearly Limited.

Van der Kolk, B.A. (1983). Psychotherapy of the elderly. General discussion: The idealizing transference and group psychotherapy with elderly patients. *Journal of Geriatric Psychiatry, 16*(1), 99–102.

Wilson, H. (1983, April). *Increased challenge for the elderly.* Paper presented at the annual convention of the Rocky Mountain Psychological Association, Snowbird, UT. (ERIC Document Reproduction Service No. 235 398)

Part II

Monthly Activities

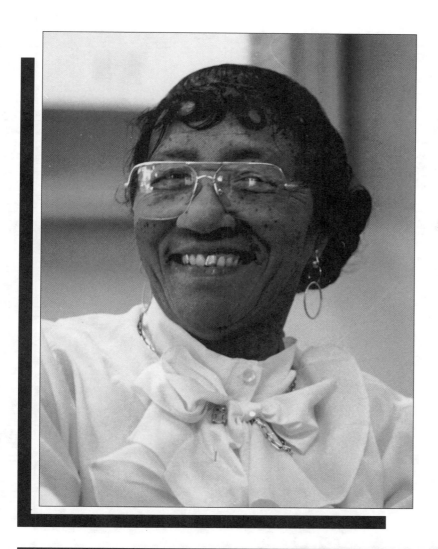

January

Themes:
Winter
Home
Health
New beginnings
Positive attitudes

New Beginnings

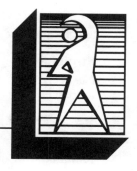

January

BEFORE

- Begin a discussion of New Year's resolutions by emphasizing the new year as a time for new beginnings.
- Suggest that one important resolution/new beginning is to improve the body's funtional capacity through movement activities.
- Direct the participants to sit in chairs that are an arm's distance apart from each other and to use correct posture.
  1. Sit up tall.
  2. Press lower back into chair.
  3. Hold abdomen in.

Warm-up

Introduce the warm-up by suggesting that participants walk away from last year's problems. Warm up for 2–3 minutes.

1. "Walk" while seated: move feet up and down; march together. Move arms back and forth.
2. Move feet apart and back together.
3. Pat hands on lap in time with feet.

Breathe

Participants who associate the removal of stress with breathing will become more relaxed. Ask the older adults to blow away old stresses from last year.

1. Breathe deeply and slowly.
2. Exhale audibly.

Stretch

Neck: Direct participants to greet their "neighbor" (the person next to them) with each turn of the neck.

1. Turn head right, left, and center; hold for 5 seconds at each turn.
2. Repeat turns 3–4 times.

Shoulders: Suggest that participants let go of last year's tension.

1. Roll shoulders to front; repeat 3–4 times.
2. Roll shoulders to back; repeat 3–4 times.

Arms/Shoulders/Back: Ask older adults to reach for the goals that they have set for the new year.

1. Reach for the ceiling, alternating arms; repeat 3–4 times.
2. Keep reaching and wiggle the fingers.

Wrists: Advise participants to think of opening the door to a brand new year while they exercise their wrists.

1. Rotate wrists forward 3–4 times.
2. Rotate wrists backward 3–4 times.

Legs: Tell participants to imagine kicking bad habits out the door while they extend their legs.

1. Alternate extending each leg 3–4 times.
2. Point and flex the feet 3–4 times.
3. Circle the foot and ankle 3–4 times.

DURING

Introduce participants to an aerobic activity that has a very low intensity level. Consider the following as a model:

1. Everyone stands and forms a large circle. (If participants are unable to stand, seated positions may be maintained with these individuals forming a circle within the circle.)
2. As the music is started, participants walk clockwise around the circle keeping time with the beat. (If seated, participants walk in place.)
3. Periodically, the leader stops the music and someone volunteers to share his or her resolution with the group. (Heart rates can be assessed at this time. Unless participants were given a graded exercise stress test, they should be instructed that their maximum heart rate should not exceed 110–120 beats per minute.)

AFTER

Ask participants to think of things they plan to do differently in the new year as they do the following cool-down.

1. Walk in place slowly for 2–3 minutes.
2. Stretch arms overhead, alternating left and right arms.
3. Raise shoulders toward ears 3–4 times.
4. Relax and give yourself a big hug.

SAFETY PRECAUTIONS

1. Encourage participants to wear flat-soled shoes to avoid slipping or turning an ankle.
2. Instruct participants to discontinue any exercise that causes pain.

Health

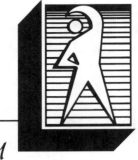

January

GOALS

- To teach participants skills that will enable them to assess their level of activity via heart rate assessment (Specifically, participants will learn to locate carotid and/or radial artery and determine heart rate. Leaders can refer to the heart rate chart and rate of perceived exertion plan in the fitness section of Chapter 3.)
- To continue to work on joint flexibility through selected stretching exercises

BEFORE

Direct participants to sit in chairs that are an arm's distance apart from each other and to use correct posture.

1. Sit up tall.
2. Press lower back into chair.
3. Hold abdomen in.

Warm-up

Prompt those participating to concentrate on all the muscles they are using as they warm up. Warm up for 2–3 minutes.

1. "Walk" while seated: move feet up and down as though marching. Move arms back and forth.
2. Move feet apart and back together.

Breathe

Instruct participants to feel their lungs expand as they inhale and listen to the sound as they exhale.

1. Breathe deeply and slowly.
2. Exhale audibly.

Stretch

Neck: Lead the participants in greeting the person next to them with each turn of the neck.

1. Turn neck right, left, and center; hold for 5 seconds at each turn.
2. Repeat 3–4 times in each direction.

Shoulders: Direct participants to loosen their upper body, an area where tension can build up.

1. Roll shoulders forward 3–4 times.
2. Roll shoulders backward 3–4 times.

Arms/Shoulders/Back: Suggest that the participants reach up and feel their arms, shoulders, and back come alive.

1. Reach for the ceiling, alternating arms 3–4 times.
2. Continue to reach upward and wiggle the fingers.

Wrists: Ask participants to loosen their hand and wrists.

1. Rotate with the right wrist 3–4 times in each direction.
2. Rotate with the left wrist 3–4 times in each direction.

Legs: Encourage participants to feel the muscles of their legs as they extend each leg. Repeat each exercise 3–4 times.

1. Alternate extending each leg.
2. Point and flex the feet alternately.
3. Circle the foot at the ankle; alternate feet.

DURING

1. Instruct the participants on how to assess their heart rate (see discussion of heart rate in Chapter 3).
   a. Demonstrate and explain how to locate the pulse at the neck, wrist, temple, and base of the heart.
   b. Encourage participants to practice locating and counting their pulse rate.
2. Explain the concept of rate of perceived exertion (see Chapter 3).
3. Introduce two modified rhythmic activities, such as the Birdie song or Hokey Pokey.

AFTER

Cool-down (perform each exercise slowly 3–4 times)

1. Roll shoulders backward.
2. Alternate turning the neck from right to left.

3. Breathe slowly and deeply.
4. Stretch the arms and shoulders (give yourself a hug).

SAFETY PRECAUTIONS

1. Have participants check their heart rate frequently to ensure that it is within the 110–120 range.
2. Make sure there is no furniture or equipment in the area where rhythmical activities take place.

Snow

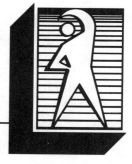

January

GOALS

- To increase joint mobility during a time of year when people are less inclined to be active.
- To keep spirits up and decrease the possibility of January depression.

BEFORE

- Ask participants to think about the snow that often falls during January. As they warm up, encourage them to think about outdoor winter activities.

- Direct participants to use correct posture. Prompt participants to think of themselves as snowmen: tall and erect.

  1. Stand (or sit) up tall.

  2. Round pelvis under, keep knees slightly bent, hold stomach in (if standing).

  3. Press lower back into chair and hold abdomen in (if seated).

Warm-up

Allow the participants to stand unless unable to do so. Suggest that they imagine shuffling through the snow while they warm up. Warm up for 2–3 minutes.

1. Walk—move feet up and down; march together—swing the arms back and forth.

2. Move feet apart and back together.

3. Extend arms out to the sides and move them up and down as if making a snow angel.

Breathe

Remind participants of how breath appears on a cold day and encourage them to imagine the shapes that their breath might make as the air comes out of their mouths.

1. Breathe deeply and slowly.
2. Exhale audibly.
3. Bring arms up with each inhalation, lower arms with each exhalation.

Stretch

Neck

1. Turn head to the right, left, and center (hold for 5 seconds at each turn); repeat 4–6 times.
2. Drop head to one shoulder, then the other (hold 5 seconds each); repeat 4–6 times.

Shoulders

1. Roll shoulders forward; repeat 4–6 times.
2. Roll shoulders backward; repeat 4–6 times.

Arms/Shoulders/Back: As the group does this exercise, suggest that they imagine snowflake trails and follow them with their arms.

1. Reach for the ceiling, alternating arms; repeat 4–6 times.
2. Continue to reach and wiggle fingers.
3. Extend arms upward and roll forward from the hips; then slowly roll back up.

Wrists: Entice group to imagine snowflakes turning in the wind as they turn their wrists.

1. Turn wrists in each direction; repeat turns 4–6 times.

Legs (while seated)

1. Alternate extending each leg; repeat 4–6 times.
2. Extend and flex the feet; repeat 4–6 times.
3. Circle each foot at the ankle; repeat 4–6 times.

Torso

1. Bring the left arm up and over the head as right hand slides down the right thigh.
2. Repeat with right arm over the head and left hand sliding down the thigh.

DURING

Engage the participants in a modified aerobic dance activity in which movements depict various activities performed when it snows. To begin, ask participants to form a large circle. Play music with a winter theme during the activity.

1. Shuffle through the snow: Using a shuffling motion with the feet, urge participants to alternate the way they move in each direction by changing the body from an upright to a semi-crouched position. Repeat moving in each direction twice.

2. Skate across the ice: By using a sliding step, stepping first on one foot and then the other, ask the group to move in a circle in each direction. Repeat a full circle 2 times.

3. Make snowballs: Direct the participants to use resistance exercises as they:

   a. Reach over and pick up a handful of snow. Press one hand into the other forming a snowball; repeat 4 times.

   b. Push hands up, out, and down; repeat 2 times with each hand.

   c. Reach out and press hands against neighbor's hands.

4. Shovel snow: Instruct the participants to make a shoveling motion first to the right and then to the left. While making the shoveling motion, step out on the right or left foot, depending on which direction the "shovel" is going; and shovel over the shoulder. Repeat 4 times in each direction.

5. Sweep the snow from the walk: Prompt the group to make a sweeping motion from side to side while stepping alternately on each foot.

AFTER

Have participants think of coming out of the snow into a nice warm room.

1. Walk in place shaking the snow from the feet.
2. Stretch arms over head to remove hat.
3. Shrug shoulders while wiggling out of a coat.
4. Lean over to untie boots.
5. Reach up, up, and up.
6. Relax and give yourself a hug.

Home-Baked Cookies

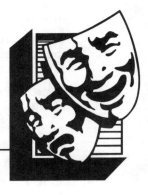

January

MATERIALS

- Ball (any size or material)
- Spoons
- Bowls
- Cookie sheets

BEFORE

1. Seat the group in a circle.
2. Toss or pass a ball to a participant.
3. Direct the person holding the ball to introduce him- or herself, name his or her favorite type of cookie, and then pass the ball to another member of the group.

The ball helps to focus attention on the participant who is speaking. This activity will encourage participants to share information and to feel more comfortable and accepting of each other.

DURING

1. Divide the group into pairs. Explain that each pair will act out skits about baking cookies. One person will play a little boy or girl and the other will be an older friend or family member. Tell the participants playing the older

friend or family member that they will be teaching the other participants how to bake cookies. Each group can opt to use the materials available. Make sure that each person understands what to do and understands that each pair will perform a skit.

2. Give each pair a few minutes to rehearse their skit before bringing the whole group together to watch the performances.

3. Encourage participants to discuss the topic shown and share experiences after each performance.

AFTER

Ask each of the participants to think of baked goods that they have made or eaten recently. Ask them if they have ever baked cookies before or helped someone bake cookies, and if so, what cookies they made, how they tasted, and what the kitchen smelled like. This discussion would be an appropriate time to offer the group some freshly baked cookies.

Expressions of Health

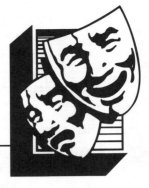

January

GOALS

- To create and perform a skit about staying healthy
- To develop an environment of trust, sharing, and cooperation
- To increase wellness skills

MATERIALS

- Chalkboard or large piece of paper or posterboard
- Beanbag, scarf, or large vitamin pill bottle

BEFORE

1. Introduce the topic of emotional and physical health and discuss the importance of the two.
2. Form the group into a circle.
3. Explain that a beanbag (or a scarf or big vitamin pill bottle) is passed within the group as a way of indicating a person's turn to speak.
4. Each person introduces himself or herself to the group and shares one way that a person can stay healthy.
5. The leader or someone acting as recorder records the responses on the board.
6. The activity continues until each person has had a chance to speak.

DURING

1. Review the responses and divide the participants into groups of three or four.
2. From the list, assign to each group one method of staying healthy.

3. Explain that each group will create a skit about that method, showing bad and good ways. For example, in a skit about food groups, it is funny to demonstrate bad food groups. Give each group a few minutes to create and rehearse their skit.

4. Assemble the entire group together and ask each group to perform.

5. Following each skit, point out the clever, funny, and original things the actors did.

AFTER

1. Review the health tips the participants offered earlier.

2. Lead a discussion of what the participants can do now to stay healthy during the next few weeks. For example, if someone has a big box of chocolates at home or in his or her room, ask what that person could do about avoiding a binge. Or, if someone mentions keeping warm, help participants think of personal strategies to deal with cold or drafty rooms, such as placing stuffed cloth "snakes" under the door.

3. Record the responses.

4. Perhaps the group would like to copy their health tips. The copies can then be handed out to friends and family.

Winter Movements

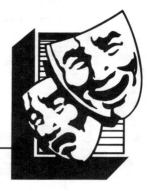

January

GOALS

- To experience the soothing quality of hand lotion
- To increase concentration levels through mirroring
- To reminisce about winter

MATERIALS

- A container of hand lotion
- Radio or cassette player and rhythmic, slow music

BEFORE

1. Instruct all participants to spread their chairs out, allowing for room.

2. Pass a container of lotion around to each person in the group, and ask them to put a dollop in their hands.

3. Have the participants talk about lotions they use in winter to keep the skin soft and moist and to avoid cracking in cold weather.

4. Beginning with hands, massage lotion into skin. Talk about how gently exercising fingers minimizes arthritis pain. Maybe some participants have some hand exercise ideas to share as well. Some participants may wish to continue to massage the lotion on their arms.

5. Inform the group that through massaging, the muscles can be warmed and stimulated.

6. Tell the group to sit straight in their chairs with their feet on the floor and their arms hanging freely by their sides. Ask participants to lace the fingers of both hands together and stretch them over their heads.

7. Ask them to name and act out a range of movements while the group follows. Urge them to recall if certain movements remind them of winter.

8. Introduce the idea of mirroring. Also, have the participants talk about good movements (to do more of) and bad movements that should be avoided or only done with caution to avoid straining the body.

DURING

1. Explain the exercise of mirroring (following one person's movements as if that person were a mirror) to the group.
2. Allow each person to select a partner. One person will be the leader and the other person will be the mirror.
3. Turn on some rhythmic, slow music.
4. Tell participants that they may use large and small movements, but that they must be in slow motion. Tell the leader of each group to select a movement that brings a winter memory, either past or present, to mind. There will be no talking allowed during this activity.
5. Remind the pairs to do their motions very slowly.
6. After a few minutes, ask the players to exchange roles. Repeat the instructions for the new leaders and begin again.

AFTER

Ask each pair to tell what movements they were making. Inquire if any of the movements seemed particularly like winter. Discuss when people remembered doing those movements in winter. Urge them to think about movement in their daily activities and if there are ways to include more good movement.

ADAPTATION

If any participants have orthopedic challenges, tell them to do only those movements that they feel comfortable doing and not to do any that seem to strain them.

Clay Sculpture

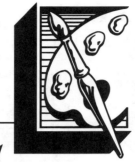

January

MATERIALS

- Low-fire clay (1 pound per person)
- Burlap squares (12" × 14")
- Newspaper or rags

BEFORE

1. Invite the group to talk about winter and their experiences with snow. Prompt them to share experiences about the *worst* winter they can recall.

2. After the discussion, ask the group to visualize lots of snow; sparkling, crisp air; frozen breath; and tree limbs drooping. Suggest that they envision the silent falling of snow.

3. Ask the group how snow crunching under their feet feels and sounds.

4. Invite the group to move as though they are shoveling snow, making snow angels, throwing snowballs, and making snow people.

DURING

1. Give everyone a soft ball of clay, about the size of a large orange, and a piece of cloth or newspaper to work on. Tell the group that by working together they are going to create a winter scene.

2. Demonstrate pinching, rolling, and squeezing clay into shapes. Suggest that some participants may want to make snowmen. Stress variations, such as large or small, skinny or fat, man or woman, girl or boy. Provide them with some ideas of what to make, such as people, sleds, trees, or animals.

3. Have a cleared space on a separate table or in the center of the work table where all of the clay sculptures can be grouped and arranged into a scene. A participant who is unable to manipulate clay could be in charge of designing the scene.

AFTER

1. When the winter scene is complete, have the participants spend a few moments looking at the overall work. Start a discussion by asking such questions as: How does this winter scene make you feel? Would you like to go to this place we have created? What would you do there? How will everyone deal with snow and ice in the real world this winter?

2. Discuss the process of working with clay. Ask participants how they rolled, pinched, and/or squeezed their clay to make this sculpture. How else might they use the movements of pinching and squeezing for the exercise of their hands.

3. If possible, take a photograph of the group sculpture.

4. Have each person put his or her own work back into a ball to be used again. Discuss how reusing clay is a form of recycling. Ask if there are other things that they use over and over again.

ADAPTATION

Participants with developmental disabilities may be more successful with a visualization exercise if they are provided with concrete images of snow scenes. Magazines and calendars are excellent resources. The public library will have a wealth of visual material that can be used.

Note: For adapting art materials for persons with severe impairments, see Anderson (1978); Clements and Clements (1984); Lindsay (1972); Ludins-Katz and Katz (1990a); and Tilley (1975) in the Suggested Readings list for art at the back of this book.

Quilt Collages

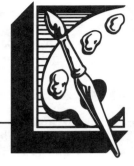

January

GOALS

- To share memories and ideas of indoor winter activities and group projects
- To work together to create something beautiful (a quilt)
- To recognize patterns in quilts and in life
- To promote manual dexterity

MATERIALS

- Scissors
- Glue
- Crayons
- Precut 8" squares of colored construction paper
- Sheets of 8½" × 11" white paper
- Large (quilt-size) piece of white butcher paper

BEFORE

1. Have the group share memories of indoor winter activities and group projects. For example, discuss quilting.
2. Examine a real quilt, if possible, or pictures of quilts. Look for patterns of shape and color.
3. Ask the group to describe their quilts or favorite quilt patterns.
4. Talk about the quilting process, for example, quilting bees and the camaraderie of this cooperative effort.

DURING

1. Distribute materials.

2. Demonstrate cutting simple geometric shapes (2" squares or triangles work well) out of white paper or distribute precut triangles and squares that participants can cut and alter.

3. Have each person arrange the shapes in a pattern on the colored construction paper square, gluing down the shapes after he or she has determined what the pattern will be. (See the adaptation note at the end of this lesson.)

4. Place colored squares on a large piece of white butcher paper that functions as a border.

5. Glue squares on in rows, creating a patchwork quilt collage.

AFTER

1. Hang the paper quilt on a wall. Invite the group to look for the patterns in the quilt collage.

2. Ask each member to find his or her square and to name the pattern he or she created. Encourage the group to identify patterns in the environment.

3. Urge participants to look around the room and to look at each other and describe the patterns on another person's clothing. For older adults who experience difficulty with this task, point out some patterns for them.

4. Discuss memories associated with quilts—warmth, sleep. Ask how much sleeping they do in cold weather as compared to warm weather. What are their sleeping patterns?

5. Have the group brainstorm places to exhibit the quilt so that many people can enjoy it. Encourage them to consider making it a group project by creating the design with fabric and auctioning the finished quilt.

ADAPTATION

Thematic quilts can be created by allowing individuals to design shapes based on seasons (winter snowflakes, snowmen, sleds, birds, trees), places (town, facility, country), or events. This provides an opportunity for older adults with exceptional visual creativity to be challenged. The group then selects one or more quilts to be sewn together in fabric. This allows any participants with sewing abilities to utilize their talent.

Making Placemats

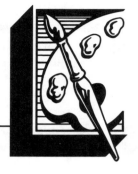

January

GOALS

- To create a placemat that illustrates a favorite healthy meal
- To look at colors and shapes of various foods
- To promote healthy eating habits
- To increase awareness of attractive table settings

MATERIALS

- Various fruits and vegetables
- Placemats
- China plate and cup
- 12" × 18" sheet of white drawing paper
- Pencils
- Water colors
- Brushes
- Reproductions of still lifes by well-known artists (available at local libraries)
- Contact paper or laminating machine (optional)

BEFORE

1. Ask the participants to discuss what foods are important in a nutritious diet. Show them a variety of fruits and vegetables.

2. Encourage the group to observe all of the foods and describe them in terms of colors and shapes.

3. Talk about the benefits of having attractive table settings. Show them placemats and china to illustrate possibilities.

4. Ask the group to share how they create a pleasant eating atmosphere in their homes.

DURING

1. Pass out white drawing paper the size of a placemat (12" × 18" is a good format).

2. With a pencil, demonstrate drawing a place setting complete with plate, utensils, napkin, cup, or glass.

3. Ask participants to think of their favorite, healthy meal and to draw an image of this delicious meal on their plate. They may want to create a border on the top and bottom of their drawing or around all of the sides.

4. After the pencil sketch is complete, distribute water colors and encourage participants to use vivid colors as they paint their drawings.

AFTER

1. Allow painting to dry. Display them on the walls or, better yet, have them laminated at a local school resource center so that they will be waterproof and can be used as placemats. (This is very inexpensive—approximately 15–40 cents per foot.) Clear contact paper can also be used as a laminating material.

2. Plan a special lunch for participants, allowing them to set a table using their own colorful paintings. The placemats can be taken home and enjoyed for months.

ADAPTATION

To adapt this lesson for persons with disabilities or dementia or for persons who do not desire to paint, photographs and/or pictures cut from magazines can be assembled into meaningful displays and laminated.

Names and Nicknames

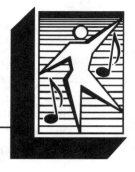

January

GOALS
• To converse with one another and get to know one another
• To feel the sense of community shared at the center or facility

BEFORE

1. Ask the participants to walk around the room and instruct them to make eye contact with the other participants, saying their own names whenever they want. The walk may vary in direction and speed.

2. Explain that when two participants meet they say their own names or each other's names and add a movement (a wave, a hop, a salute, etc.). They continue to move together, then part and walk until they join someone else.

3. Participants should try to use the space fully so that "duets" (the encounters between two people) do not all occur in the center of the room.

DURING

1. The dancers stand in a circle and consider a nickname for one participant at a time; they should come up with nicknames that sound like the participant's name. The nicknames should be real words; for example, "Joyce" might inspire the nickname of "juice," "joyous," or "choice." Everyone should have a turn to receive a nickname. The nicknames may suggest a mood or style of movement. "Heather's" nickname of "Feather," for example, might inspire floating, wispy, or even sharp quill-like movements. "Joyce's" nickname of "Choice" might inspire very indecisive movement that changes direction.

2. Introduce each member of the group and his or her new name and direct the group to move in a manner suggested by each participant's nickname.

AFTER

1. Begin a group discussion by asking each of the participants questions concerning how it felt to meet new people this week, what nicknames they received or gave to members of the group, and what they learned from this activity.

2. Ask the adults to take a minute to say good-bye to each other before they leave.

3. Thank them for their participation by complimenting them on their spirit and type of participation.

ADAPTATION

This lesson can be adapted to include people who cannot hear by giving the whole group (those with and without hearing impairments) nametags. Instruct everyone to write his or her name on one nametag and stick it on his or her shirt. Stick several blank nametags on as well. During the "naming" sequence, provide everyone with markers and instruct them to write the nickname directly on one of the person's blank nametags. When every nametag contains a name, the group is ready to begin creating movements.

Snow Sculpting

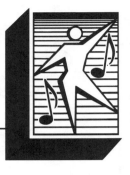

January

GOALS

- To enjoy a mock snowball fight
- To engage upper bodies and isolate individual body parts
- To catalyze group interaction
- To stimulate memories of past winter fun
- To notice how certain body postures convey different attitudes (e.g., shy postures, confident postures, direct postures, confused postures)

MATERIALS

- A large quantity of newspaper
- A large box
- Cassette player
- Music with a snow theme (e.g., "Let it Snow," "Snowy Morning Blues")

BEFORE

1. Invite participants to crumple up enough newspaper "snowballs" for a decent snowball fight.
2. If participants did not do a fitness activity immediately before this one, have them warm up as described in the dance section of Chapter 3 in Part 1 of this book while playing music with a snow theme.

DURING

1. Invite participants to form a circle.
2. Make sure everyone has an ample supply of "snowballs."

3. Let the snowball fight begin. If the group seems reluctant, feel free as the leader to toss the first few "snowballs" yourself.

4. You might want to walk around the room stuffing "snow" down a few backs. Generally, prompt them to participate.

5. When the newspaper runs out, have the group mime the action. People can play pantomime catch back and forth, or can mime throwing and being hit. During both phases of the "fight," call out different movement commands such as "Freeze!", "Slow Motion!", "Double Time!", "Jerky!", "Straight arms and legs!", or others the leader or participants can invent.

AFTER

1. Bring the snowball fight to a close.

2. Instruct participants to collect the "snow" and place it in a box in the center of the room. The newspaper can then be recycled; snow, after all (as water) is recycled.

Bringing Art to Life

January

MATERIALS

- Original art or reproductions of art with several people as part of the subject
- Easel, a stand, or some other way to display the art (e.g., tape)

BEFORE

1. Introduce this week's activity by beginning a group discussion with general questions about dance. Ask where in the community one can see dance and/or movement, and where each participant has been, is going, or would like to go, for advance experience.

2. Discuss the concept of being surrounded by movement and dance. Review by name some of the places that the group cited for dance and movement. Introduce another place to find dance and movement in art.

3. Direct the group's attention to the work of art displayed. Ask the group to share what they see in the displayed art. The leader should record the participants' responses for later use. Inquire how the painting makes them feel, what the painting reminds them of, how that memory makes them feel, what they think the story behind the painting is, what they think happened right before the scene depicted in the painting, and what they think happened right after.

DURING

1. Divide the participants into groups with the same number of people as are in the painting.
2. Instruct each group to come up with a series of movements to bring the painting to life telling what happened right after the moment captured in the painting.
3. Allow a few minutes to choreograph their routines.
4. Bring the groups together. Allow adequate time for each group to perform their routine.

AFTER

1. Gather in a circle. Begin a discussion by asking each of the groups such questions as:
    -   Where have you seen a painting that reminded you of something else?
    -   Where else can you find paintings and/or prints?
    -   How has this activity helped you to understand the story in a painting?
    -   How can you apply this lesson to everyday life?
2. Thank each of the participants for his or her participation. Give recognition for jobs well done.
3. Advise the participants that as they go through the week they should remember that things are not always as they seem. Convey the idea that what we see is a snapshot and that we create the beginning and the ending (or the context used to give it meaning).

ADAPTATION

When people with visual impairments are part of the group, instruct participants with sight to describe the painting in close detail. Suggest that the persons with the impairment ask questions about the art. Once everyone is satisfied that the painting, sculpture, or print has been communicated, proceed with the lesson. Speculation on what could happen before or after the scene in the work is then possible for those who are blind.

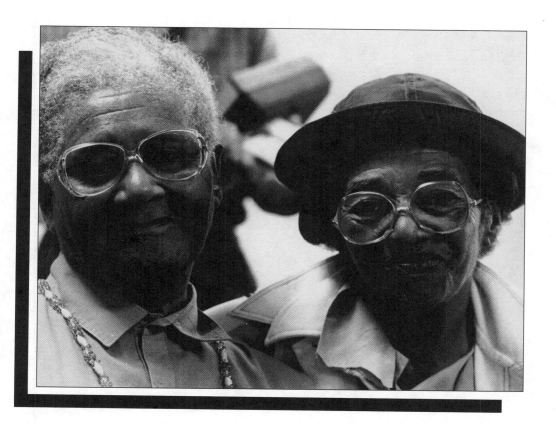

February

Themes:

Friendship
Communication
Love
Brotherhood
Sisterhood
Goodwill

Valentine's Day Party

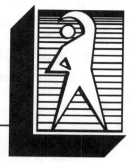

February

GOALS

- To increase strength and flexibility through stretching and movement activities
- To improve cardiorespiratory endurance through rhythmical activity

MATERIALS

- Cassette player
- Music with a romantic theme (e.g., "Love Is Blue")
- Red and pink construction paper
- Scissors

BEFORE

- Remind participants that it is February and ask them to share what comes to mind when they think about this specific time of year.
- Mention Valentine's Day and elaborate on the types of events and behaviors that occur on this date (e.g., exchanging Valentines, sending or receiving candy, sending or receiving flowers, Valentine's Day parties).
- Ask the group to divide into two lines with participants standing (if possible) and facing each other.
- Suggest that caring for someone makes a person feel very tall. Direct participants to use correct posture.
  1. Walk (or roll) to center and face your partner.
  2. Stand tall, knees slightly bent (or sit up straight, shoulders back).
  3. Round pelvis under.

Warm-up

Narrate a story that tells of members of the group arriving at a Valentine's Day party. Create a scene in which they spot someone who is special to them. Warm up for 2–3 minutes.

1. Walk toward each other and then walk backward to original position. Repeat 2 times.
2. Repeat and clap hands with partner. Repeat 2 times.
3. Walk toward partner, clap hands with partner, and pull through to the other side.
4. Walk toward partner, pull through, and return to original position.

Breathe

Remind the group of how a special person can make one breathe a little faster. Suggest that they practice breathing slowly.

1.· With hands on hips, inhale slowly and exhale slowly. Repeat 2 times.
2. With hands at sides, inhale and raise arms out to the side and then overhead.
3. Exhale and lower the arms to the sides.

Stretch

Neck: Invite participants to look in both directions to see if others are in pairs.

1. Turn right, left, and center; hold in each direction for 5 seconds.
2. Repeat neck turns in each direction 3–4 times.

Shoulders: Suggest that while mirroring their partner, each participant makes a flirtatious gesture.

1. Roll right shoulder back. Repeat 4 times.
2. Roll left shoulder back. Repeat 4 times.

Arms/Shoulders/Back: During this exercise, instruct group members to beckon their partner to come closer.

1. Alternate arm swings forward and down. Repeat 4 times with each arm.
2. Pull left arm across body by grasping at the elbow with the right hand. Repeat 4 times. Repeat with the right arm 4 times. Hold 5–10 seconds each time.
3. With a partner, make a "bridge" with arms over head. Continuing to face partner, stretch arms out to sides. Repeat 4 times.
4. Stretch arms high overhead and slowly roll forward on toes. Repeat 4 times.

DURING

- Ask the group what song best represents their understanding of romantic love.
- Suggest music, such as "Love Is Blue," for the following exercise.

Rhythmical activity: Musical Hearts (similar to Musical Chairs)

1. Cut out hearts and place them 2–3 feet apart on the floor in a circle.
2. Tell the group to begin moving counter-clockwise in a circle as the music begins to play. When the music stops (leader stops music periodically), participants must make sure they are standing on a heart.

Modified aerobic dance: Suggest that the group imagine that the Valentine's dance is about to begin. Play music such as "My Funny Valentine."

1. Have the group form a large circle.
2. Step to the right together. Continue moving right and add a big arm circle with the right arm.
3. Repeat the movements to the left.
4. Stand in place and circle the right arm and then the left arm. Repeat and circle arms in the opposite direction.
5. Step to the right 2 times, then to the left 2 times. Move right heel out, then left heel. March 4 steps in place. Repeat the sequence 4 times.
6. Continue with the above sequence and add arm movements. Push arms out to the right 2 times, to the left 2 times, and to the front 2 times. Circle arms all the way around while marching 4 steps. Repeat until music stops.

An alternate to the above suggestion is to make up a modified aerobic dance to go with music.

AFTER

- Tell the group that the party is over.
- Tell participants to begin saying good-night.
- Ask participants to think about what they like most about Valentine's Day.
  1. Walk slowly around the circle moving in a clockwise direction. Turn and walk in the opposite direction.
  2. Facing the center of the circle, reach up with one hand and then the other. Make a waving motion while hand is in the air.
  3. Give yourself a big hug, simulating a hug given to a sweetheart or spouse.

SAFETY PRECAUTIONS

Caution participants not to move too quickly during the rhythmical activity when they are standing on a paper heart.

A Friend Is Someone Who Loves You

GOALS

- To develop an appreciation of physical activity
- To appreciate the role of friendship

BEFORE

- Ask the group to think about the importance of friendship and how the love of a friend has enriched their lives.
- Motivate participants to improve their posture by reminding them that being a friend to someone makes a person feel taller.
    1. Form a circle.
    2. Facing the center of the circle, stand tall with knees slightly bent and pelvis rounded under (or sit up straight with shoulders back).
    3. Concentrate on trying to align body parts.

Warm-up

Suggest to the group that having a good friend makes us feel special.

1. Walk in a circle, carefully swinging arms back and forth. Hold head high and stretch the body upright. Repeat 2 times.
2. Turn and face the other direction and walk in a circle for 6 steps, then walk 6 steps on tip-toe.

Breathe

Engage the group in breathing exercises by stating that having someone to care for and someone who returns affection makes one breathe easier.

1. With hands on hips, inhale and exhale. Repeat 2 times.
2. With hands at sides, inhale and raise arms out to the sides and then overhead. Exhale and lower the arms back to the sides.

Stretch

Neck: Suggest that participants greet the person to each side of them as if seeing a close friend for the first time in a long while.

1. Turn head right, left, and center; hold for 5 seconds in each direction.
2. Repeat neck turns in each direction 4–6 times.

Arms/Shoulders: Inform the group that when they apologize to a friend they just shrug it off because friends easily forgive.

1. Raise shoulders and hold for 5 seconds before relaxing; repeat 2 times.
2. Raise shoulders alternately, first right then left. Hold for 3 seconds; repeat 2 times.

Arms/Shoulders/Back: Remind the group that doing something with a friend is always more fun than doing it alone.

1. With a partner, make a "bridge" with arms extended overhead (mirror partner). Stretch arms out to the sides, then over the head again. Repeat 4 times.
2. Pull left arm across body by grasping at the elbow with the right hand. Hold for 5 seconds. Repeat with right arm.

Hands/Fingers: Suggest that as the group exercises their hands, they count the many things they have shared with a friend.

1. Gently press the tip of each finger against the thumb. Go back and forth with the four fingers.
2. Repeat each finger several times.

Hips/Legs

1. Stand and hold on to a support. Extend one leg backward, keeping it straight; hold for 5 seconds. Repeat 4 times.
2. Stand and hold on to a support and perform ankle circles with the right foot, then the left foot. Repeat 4 times.

DURING

Introduce the main activity by acquainting the group with the idea that friends double our joy and divide our grief. Divide the group into two lines facing each other.

1. Walk forward and meet the person in the same position in the opposite line, then walk back again.
2. Repeat and clap hands with the person.
3. Repeat and clasp right hands and pull through to opposite side.
4. Repeat and pull through to original side.
5. Walk toward each other and make a "bridge" with arms stretched overhead.
6. Turn with partner and face same direction. Walk in a circle around the room side by side with partner.
7. When a walk around the circle is complete, face the center of the circle.

8. Step together on right foot (forward). Step together on left foot (forward).

9. Step together with right foot to the right, then with left foot to the left.

10. Bring arms upward in front of body, out to the sides and down.

AFTER

Ask the participants to think back about some of their best friends. What made them so special? Why did they make them feel so special?

1. Extend arms overhead, stretch left, then right. Repeat 3–4 times. As the stretches are repeated, step left, then right.

2. Drop one hand behind back and give yourself a pat on the back. Repeat with opposite arm and hand.

3. Bring both arms around your body and give yourself a hug.

4. End the session by giving hugs and/or pats on the back to "friends."

Winter's Last Blast

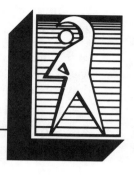

February

GOALS

- To improve balance and increase flexibility
- To make the best of cold weather

MATERIALS

- Cassette player and cassettes

BEFORE

- Introduce this topic by asking when winter's last cold blast will occur.
- Continue the theme of the lesson by discussing posture in relation to cold weather. For example, discuss how it is difficult to relax and stand up tall when shivering
  1. Stand up straight and try to align body parts.
  2. Tighten abdomen.

Warm-up

Suggest to the group that the last week in February usually brings the last of the very cold weather. Inspire participants to move by mentioning that one way to beat the cold is to get the body warm through physical activity.

1. Walk briskly in single file around the room. (To work on balance, strips of tape may be placed on the floor at various points and participants can be encouraged to walk on the tape.)
2. Continue to walk, forming a circle. Alternate walking on heels and toes.
3. When the circle is complete, walk in place while swinging arms.

Breathe

Engage the group in breathing exercises by encouraging them to visualize their breath as steam; in cold weather, their breath is visible.

1. Inhale slowly (repeat 5 times).
2. Exhale slowly.

Stretch

Neck: Suggest that participants pantomime tying a scarf around their neck as they rotate their head.

1. Turn head to the right and hold 5 seconds.
2. Turn head to the left and hold 5 seconds.
3. Repeat turning in each direction 5–6 times.

Shoulders: Lead the group in shrugging the shoulders as a carefree response to the cold weather.

1. Stand with back straight.
2. Slowly raise shoulders as high as possible in an exaggerated shrug and hold 5 seconds.
3. Return to original position.
4. Repeat 5–6 times.

Arms: Challenge the group to shake the chill with a few vigorous movements of the arms.

1. Extend arms out to the sides.
2. Make small circles behind back with arms and hands 5–6 times.
3. Repeat circle movement with arms in front of the body.

Wrists: Remind the group that one way to keep the hands warm is to rub them together.

1. Hold right wrist in left hand and rotate right wrist 5–6 times.
2. Repeat with the left wrist and right hand.

Torso: Suggest that a few calisthenics will combat the cold.

1. Stand with feet shoulder-width apart with legs straight.
2. Let one arm hang to side, extend the other arm over the head.
3. Bend slowly toward the side with the arm hanging down and stretch as far as is comfortable.
4. Return to upright position.
5. Repeat stretching to opposite side.
6. Stretch 5–6 times to each side.

Legs: Suggest that vigorous movements will help heat the body.

1. Sitting in a chair with feet on the floor, straighten the right leg out in front of chair. Bend right knee and return the foot to the floor. Repeat 5–6 times.
2. Repeat 5–6 times with the left leg.

Ankles: Direct the group to stimulate the circulation in cold feet.

1. Sitting in a chair with feet on the floor, flex and extend the right foot 5–6 times.
2. Repeat with left foot.

DURING

1. Ask participants to stand in a scattered formation.
2. Select music with an uplifting beat and a winter theme.
3. Advise participants to think of a cold, blustery day and of the many routine things they do on such a day, such as putting on a coat, walking briskly, throwing wood on the fire, and lifting their feet alternately off the floor to stimulate circulation.
4. As the music begins, direct participants to move to the beat of the music, moving in ways that demonstrate winter activities. Any movement that reminds them of winter is acceptable—the important thing is to keep moving.
5. Repeat an aerobic activity from one of the previous fitness lessons.

AFTER

Tell the group that winter is coming to a close. Ask them to think of the warm sun, being able to move at a slower pace and not be cold, and the beginning of spring.

1. Walk slowly around the room.
2. Slowly swing both arms to the left and overhead, then to the right and down forming a big circle. Repeat 3–5 times.
3. Repeat circular movements in opposite direction.
4. Breathe in and out slowly.

Enacting Stories About Unrequited Love

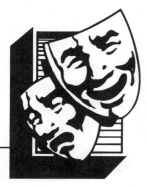

February

BEFORE

1. Clip sentences or paragraphs of a love story from a novel or a ladies' magazine.
2. Select sentences or paragraphs that the group would be comfortable acting out and that include action.
3. Spread the pieces of paper out on a table.
4. Have participants pick up pieces and read aloud the sentences or episodes that interest them.

DURING

1. Any shy participants should be prompted to give the leader one of the sentences to act out, in order to show the group what fun this activity can be.
2. After the leader finishes, participants select one of the episodes to act out or to discuss. The may pair up with a buddy to make the selection and perform the part.

AFTER

1. Share a time in your life when your affection for another person was not reciprocated. Tell of silly, funny things you did that you can laugh about now.
2. Encourage participants to share such episodes from their lives and from their present situations.

Why We Are Lovable

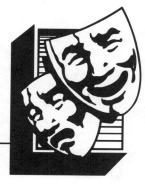

February

MATERIALS

- Personal ads seeking companionship that include a list of the seeker's positive characteristics.

BEFORE

1. Begin a discussion about the worth of people as individuals
2. Discuss how sometimes people forget how valuable or lovable they are
3. Tell the following story: "A wise old Greek named Socrates used to wander the streets of Athens saying 'Know thyself.' He had learned that if people did not understand themselves, they probably could not understand other people."
4. Discuss how understanding ourselves is not easy and that our total self is the combination of many parts. These parts include:

   Physical self, which includes body skills and physical characteristics, such as weight, height, age, color of eyes and hair, and so forth

   Psychological self, which includes feelings, emotions, values, and personality traits

   Social self, which includes how individuals act and feel with others

DURING

1. Ask the group to divide into pairs or small groups.

2. Have the participants read personal ads from the daily paper or some other source. Depending on the source of advertisements, it may be prudent to screen the selections to avoid offending anyone.

3. To model the activity, ask the group to assist you in writing an advertisement for yourself.

4. Have the participants develop a personal ad for each of the persons in their group. Be sure that the individual agrees with the qualities listed. Encourage participants to include all three aspects of a person: physical, psychological, and social.

5. A humorous variation on this theme is also to have the participants list the characteristics desired in a person being sought.

AFTER

The results of this activity can be shared in several ways. They can be read aloud to the group by the participant, a friend, or the leader. Appreciative discussion confirming that person's strengths should occur before going on to the next participant. The statements can be written up as a record of the strengths, achievements, and interests of the participants. They could be used on a "Person of the Day" bulletin board, which might also include a "Person of Tomorrow." This bulletin board might spur thinking of special ways to recognize that person as unique on his or her day; for example, the singing of a song about roses for a person with the name of Rose.

Valentine Candy Fortunes

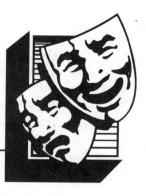

February

GOALS
- To have fun
- To relate to other people

MATERIALS

- A box of Valentine heart candies in pastel colors with words of endearment printed on them; approximately five pieces for each participant
- Chalkboard and large piece of paper

BEFORE

1. Give each participant five or more pieces of the candy.
2. Ask each participant to read some of his or her favorite phrases aloud to the group.
3. Using a chalkboard or a large piece of paper, write out some of the phrases for other participants to see.

DURING

1. Have the participants form circles of about five people.
2. Each participant distributes his or her pieces of candy to the individuals he or she thinks best fit that description. All of the candies should be distributed.
3. Each person reads to the group the Valentine heart characteristics that were given to him or her. The person states whether the characteristics do or do not accurately describe his or her personality, and whether some other good trait was inadvertently overlooked.

4. Participants may wish to play a second round of this game, forming new groups and redistributing the candies to others.

AFTER

1. With the group assembled, and using a chalkboard or large sheet of paper, decide if there were some traits that were omitted from the standard ones on the Valentine candies, and which sayings the group could playfully suggest for inclusion on next year's candy printing.

2. As a way of wrapping up the lesson on a more serious note, discuss what characteristics were pointed out today that everyone could benefit from each day.

ADAPTATION

For individuals with challenges in reading, the leader, a friend, or a helper can read the messages to the person and/or use body movements to convey the idea. The individual who does not speak can show through body movements or a communication board with symbols and/or words or letters, depending on the level of the individual, what he or she wants to communicate.

Collage from Magazine Photos

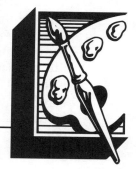

February

GOALS

- To create a collage of loving people and loving deeds
- To share feelings about friends and loved ones
- To identify important people in the lives of the participants
- To focus on positive actions that show the love of others
- To improve manual dexterity and flexibility

MATERIALS

- Magazines
- Scissors
- Glue
- Oil pastels
- Rulers
- 12" × 18" sheets of colored construction paper

BEFORE

Initiate a discussion about different people who are or were important in the participants' lives by asking such questions as: Who are some people who have been special in your life? What things did those people do to show you they cared for you? How did they make you feel loved? What do you do today to make someone's day a little brighter? What are things you can do to be helpful to others?

DURING

1. Distribute collage materials.
2. Ask group members to work with a partner.

3. Instruct participants to cut or tear out pictures from old magazines that remind them of people who have cared for them, and people or pets for whom they care. Include pictures of people doing loving things for others.

4. Tell participants to use a pencil and a ruler to draw a 1½" border around the edges of the colored sheet of construction paper, and to go over the pencil line with oil pastel to create a rectangle.

5. Participants glue the magazine cutouts in the center rectangle of the paper, filling the space and bumping the inner edges of the border. Be sure to glue images on carefully, smoothing down all of the edges.

6. Participants design a colorful border around the edges of the collage using oil pastels. A symbol of love, such as a heart, could be repeated to create an interesting border pattern.

AFTER

1. Display the collages around the room as a stimulus to discuss giving love and showing affection. This could also be a time to talk about the opposite emotions of feeling useless and unloved.

2. Make a list of strategies for coping with unpleasant situations and share how participants have successfully used these strategies.

3. Talk about being gracious and forgiving to all people, no matter how much we may or may not like them.

4. Collages can be laminated at a nearby school or media center and used for placemats that participants can enjoy all year.

Body Language –
Creating Clay Figures

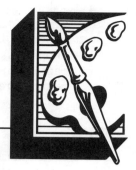

February

GOALS

- To create clay figures expressive of emotion
- To focus on building friendships
- To discuss the importance of communication
- To examine different ways of communicating

MATERIALS

- Table for clay work
- One pound of low-fire clay per person
- Canvas or burlap squares
- Plastic knives
- Toothpicks
- Moistened sponges or paper towels
- Shallow containers
- Hand lotion
- Illustrations of sculptures of human figures

BEFORE

1. Have participants form a circle.
2. Begin a discussion of friendship. Encourage the group to share their feelings about special friends in their lives. Prompt a dialogue about what makes a good friendship and the importance of communicating thoughts and feelings to each other.

3. Ask participants how they let one another know what they are thinking and feeling, and if there is a way they can let someone know how they are feeling without putting it into words.

4. Ask the group to "act out" feelings through gestures, posture, facial expressions, and so forth (e.g., drooping shoulders can indicate sadness or fatigue, hands on hips can mean frustration or anger, arms uplifted could mean happiness). Let the activity take on a game-like approach. Participants can pantomime feelings while the rest of the group tries to guess what feeling is being expressed.

DURING

1. Distribute canvas or burlap squares and a grapefruit-size ball of low-fire clay to each participant.

2. Pinch off some of the clay and demonstrate forming a figure by shaping the clay into a log or roll about 4–5 inches long.

3. Using a plastic knife, cut about one third of the way up the middle of the log. This will create the legs of the figure. Pinch out a head and neck shape at the top of the form. Arms can be added by rolling out a coil of clay and attaching it to the back of the figure, smoothing it until it looks like a part of the original clay body.

4. Once participants assemble their figures, suggest that they experiment with different poses and gestures. Ask group members to decide what feelings they want their sculpture to express. They can manipulate the clay until they are satisfied with the message the figure is conveying.

AFTER

1. Place clay sculptures in the center of the table and have participants look at all of them. How successful was the group in using body language? Did more than one participant try to communicate the same feeling in their sculpture? Did they use similar gestures?

2. Have participants pantomime the movements in each other's artwork and guess to whose art the performance refers.

3. Store clay sculptures in a safe place and allow them to dry for about 10 days before firing. It may be difficult to gain access to a kiln for firing. Good resources are local art centers, art teachers at nearby schools, or potters who have studios in the area. If it is not possible to fire the clay, do not be discouraged—clay can be recycled easily. Take a photograph of the group's work, ball the clay back up, mist it with water, and store it in a plastic bag to be used again.

ADAPTATION

For persons with visual impairments, provide added verbal and physical rein-
forcements in preparation of making sculpture. During the "before" or "during"
activities, encourage persons with limited vision to portray a feeling and to be
especially aware of the stresses and strains they feel on their body while doing
the portrayal. For example, with an arm curled around another's shoulder, stress
can be felt on the shoulder, back, and on the corresponding leg. Encourage the
group to ask the actor questions about how and where the stresses are felt and to
guess the feeling while at the same time giving verbal feedback on how the action
appears.

A Musical Painting

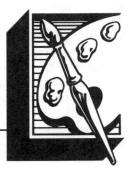

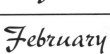
February

GOALS

- To make a "music painting"
- To enhance and integrate a sense of sight and a sense of sound
- To increase appreciation and recognition of African-American music

MATERIALS

- Cassette player
- Cassettes of African-American music (spirituals, gospel, blues, jazz)
- Large white drawing paper or newsprint (at least 18" × 24")
- Markers or tempera paint and brushes

BEFORE

1. Point out great contributions African-American musicians make and have made to American culture.

2. Play examples of African-American music; if there are lyrics, have the group discuss the meaning of the words. What kinds of themes or domains does the music tap? Is the music in the realm of the spiritual, intellectual, or emotional domains? Is the music about lost love?

3. Have participants move in rhythm to the music. If they can, have them clap, tap their feet, or use their entire body.

4. Ask participants to share a favorite song and start a group "sing-a-long."

DURING

1. Give each participant a large piece of white drawing paper and paint, markers, or crayons.

2. Play the tape once again and ask the group to paint or draw as they listen to the music, making marks based on what they hear.

3. Encourage them to let their hands simply respond to the rhythm in the music. (If space is available, a very large piece of butcher paper can be affixed to the wall and participants can use their entire bodies to respond rhythmically as they draw.)

AFTER

Display the musical paintings or drawings on the walls. Have the group look closely for linear patterns that mirror rhythmic patterns in the music. Is there a difference in the way the line moves depending on the tempo of the music?

This lesson could be expanded into a week of listening to music of other cultures. Prompt a discussion by asking such questions as: Have you ever listened to music of the Far East, Native America, or India? What other types of music would be fun to listen and paint to? Does anyone have a tape they would like to bring and share with others?

An excellent 80-minute video, "Say Amen Somebody," offers a wonderful glimpse into the world of the African-American gospel tradition. The film features octogenarians Thomas Dorsey and Willie Mae Ford Smith, early gospel singers who give dynamic performances that guarantee viewers a toe-tapping, hand-clapping experience. If possible, this video could be shown to participants to provide them with more information about African-American music.

Communicating Through Body Language

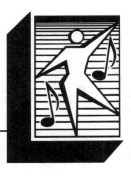

February

GOALS

- To develop the concentration and attentiveness required to move in unison with another person and to experience the bonding and trust created by shared leadership
- To enjoy seeing how all people "speak" their own movement "language"—a chance to see how one's movement can tell a story without using verbal language
- To expand "movement vocabularies" by performing the movement of others

---

BEFORE

1. If the group did not do a fitness activity immediately before this lesson, do the basic warm-up described in the Dance section of Chapter 3, this volume.

2. Introduce mirroring. This exercise works best when participants are in a calm, quiet mood, so it may be appropriate to begin the session with a short progressive relaxation to quiet everyone down.

3. Direct partners to sit quietly in chairs facing each other and begin by breathing together. Slowly, one partner begins to move and the other mirrors his or her movements as exactly as possible. This means that "unintentional" movements (yawning, blinking, laughing) are mirrored just like any other. Partners should not talk at any time, but must pay close attention to each other. The goal of this exercise is for partners to feel that they are moving as if they are one being. With some practice, they should not be able to tell who is leading and who is following. This is a very exciting moment! Demonstrate with a partner, emphasizing slow movement, strong focus, and close unison.

DURING

1. Have participants pair up again, perhaps with different partners.

2. Partner A begins making a movement, any movement. Partner B imitates that movement and responds with one of his or her own. Partner A then imitates Partner B's response and adds a new movement of his or her own.

3. Let these duets go on for a few minutes, then have the group split in half and let one half watch the other. Switch to observing the other half of the group.

4. Notice how different duets have different qualities. Some "conversations" may be slow and serious, others light and playful. Discuss how the movement choices give these impressions.

5. Try this same activity with groups of five to eight members, depending on memory abilities. One person begins with a movement. The next person repeats the first person's movement and adds on of his or her own. The third person repeats movements 1 and 2 and adds a movement, and so forth until everyone has contributed a movement.

6. Ask the group to repeat the sequence a few times; when all participants feel confident that they know it, let them show it to the other group.

7. This activity can be varied by having people imitate exactly what the person just before them did (rather than how the movement was done originally), so that people's "mistakes" are incorporated into the phrase. This version is similar to the game "Telephone."

AFTER

1. Form a circle and discuss what participants saw and felt. How are movements "telling"? Did different "movement personalities" emerge? How did partners choose to respond to each other? How did it feel to "talk" this way? Were people able to "say" what they wanted to? What did participants notice about how movements changed going from one body to another? Were individual variations sometimes just as pleasing to watch as the original movement?

2. Suggest that participants watch for mirroring throughout the week. Attitudinal similarities and differences can be evidenced in the way people move in relation to each other. Have them look for real-life situations. For example, when one person sits down, does the other sit down soon afterward? How do people mirror each other when they talk? How does mirroring reflect agreement or disagreement?

3. Suggest that participants use mirroring in everyday situations.

Note

When people are in agreement with each other or concentrating on what a person has to say, they tend to mirror the other person. Thus, they face each other directly, sit when the other person is sitting, nod heads with each other, and laugh simultaneously. In conversation, they tend to mirror each other by recapping the statements made by the other person. This is a very sophisticated way of ensuring that one is heard by the other person and acknowledging the importance of the other person's ideas. However, when people disagree or are threatening one another, they tend to use body language contrary to the other person's. They tend to turn away, respond with silence, not make eye contact, have their arms folded, and generally not acknowledge the other person's statements or presence. This mode of behavior tends to make people feel threatened or hostile and is not productive for problem solving, Thus, attention to mirroring can aid in communication and in constructing positive relationships.

Connections

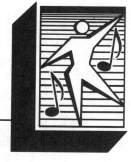

February

> ## GOALS
>
> - To refine mirroring skills and experience shared leadership
> - To experience the different kinds of shapes the body can make
> - To respond to and connect with others through shape and movement
> - To develop cooperative and collaborative skills by sharing in a creative process

MATERIALS

- Polaroid camera (optional)

BEFORE

1. If the group did not do a fitness activity before this lesson, do the basic warm-up described in the Dance section of Chapter 3.

2. Have the group divide into pairs and do about 5–10 minutes of mirroring. Let them begin without a designated leader, but with leadership passing back and forth.

3. Reconvene the group and share experiences. How does this feel different from the last time they experienced mirroring? When and where have they noticed mirroring during the course of their lives?

DURING

1. Have the group divide into pairs with new partners. Have Partner A make a shape and hold it. (The shape could be one of radiating limbs, of a curve, or of sharp angles.) Partner B then makes a shape that connects with partner A. Direct partners to remember this shape.

2. Let Partner A make another shape and let Partner B make a new connecting shape. Tell them to remember this shape well.

3. Direct the pairs to make two more connecting shapes, this time with Partner B beginning. Let them rehearse the sequence of four shapes.

4. Have the pairs show their shapes to the group.

5. To continue this exercise, have the partners connect their four shapes with movements, so that one shape flows into the next in a dance phrase. These phrases can be rehearsed until partners are confident that they remember them and can show them to the group.

6. Tell everyone to move to the edges of the room. To begin this activity, one person goes to the center of the room and makes a shape with his or her body. Another person joins the first person, making a shape that connects with the first person's in some way. One by one let people come into the center of the circle and connect with at least one other person.

7. Encourage participants to explore the different ways there are to connect with each other. For instance, they can connect by linking body parts, by touching, or by intersecting. When everyone has joined in, the result is a giant group shape.

8. Divide the group in half, let one half watch the other, and then switch. If balance is a problem, participants may sit or hold on to chairs. If participants cannot hold their shapes long enough for the entire group to join in the shape, work in smaller groups.

9. If a camera is available, take pictures of each "human sculpture."

AFTER

1. Ask the group to share experiences and observations. Center the discussion on the shapes the participants noticed while doing the activity.

2. Expand the discussion to relevant shapes observed in the community. Responses might include church steeples that are long and pointed, doors that are rectangular in shape, pools that are circular. Discuss the most common shapes found and why.

3. Ask participants to describe the most unusual shapes they have seen.

4. If applicable, display the photographs taken of the group while they were doing the "connections." Apply the same patterns of discussion used above to the photos.

ADAPTATION

Consider the abilities of the members of your group when deciding the number of shapes you direct them to create and remember. Persons with developmental disabilities may be able to remember only one or two shapes, whereas other older adults may remember up to eight. (Short-term memory usually holds between seven and nine items.) Persons with severe dementia may require modeling or actual placement. Positive experiences during the process are of prime importance. Challenge everyone according to his or her capacity.

So Far Away

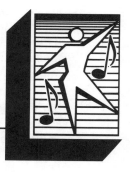

February

GOALS

- To provide an opportunity for spontaneous expression of feelings
- To increase daily level of physical activity

BEFORE

1. Have participants do the basic warm-up described in the Dance section of Chapter 3.

2. Stimulate a discussion about people who are a part of the participants' lives, but are not able to be close to them. Discuss the meaning each person has to them and the major attributes of the person.

3. Let each participant pick at least four people who are far away.

DURING

1. Ask participants to make four movements that represent the four people they chose.

2. Direct each participant to put the movements together while adding four movements that represent his or her own self.

3. Suggest that they alternate the movements, one of theirs and one that they have attributed to someone else, and that they continue to do this until they have eight moves together.

4. Remind the group to use as many parts of their bodies as possible; suggest that they dance with their feet, their hands, their necks, and so forth.

5. Rehearse the movements with the participants in slow motion, then faster.

6. Suggest that they perform their individual dances for each other.

AFTER

1. Begin a group discussion by asking each of the participants to discuss one of the people they chose—someone who lives far away and whom they care about. Ask them to share just how they feel when they are away from them. Do their loved ones know how they feel about being separated from them? If the answer is yes, ask them to share their technique in communicating those feelings. If the answer is no, elicit from the group ways of expressing to a loved one feelings of this nature.

2. Ask participants to share some things that can be done to feel close to people who are missed and are far away. Suggest that those with loved ones far away try using some of the suggestions and techniques revealed in the dance experience.

ADAPTATION

Instruct people who have limited or no use of their arms or legs to create facial expressions to represent people whom they care about and are far away. Other expressions could represent themselves. Suggest that they differentiate the expressions by turning their necks or their wheelchairs in one direction for the expressions relating to others and another direction for those relating to themselves.

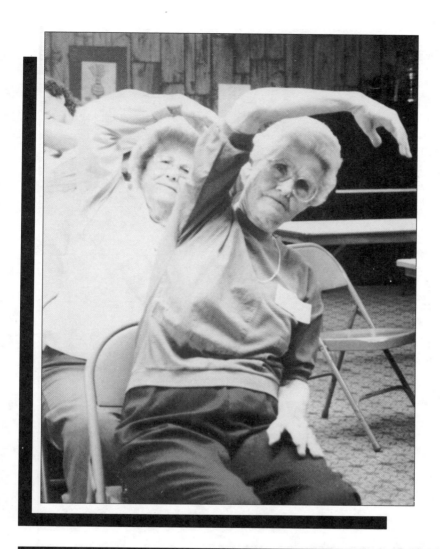

March

Themes:
Wind and weather
Joy
Happiness
Pleasure
Delight
A positive outlook

Flying in the Wind

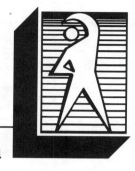

March

GOALS

- To strengthen participants' upper bodies through exercise
- To evoke memories of kite flying
- To develop the capacity to respond to the imagination

MATERIALS

- Cassette player and cassettes

BEFORE

- Inform the group that to fly a kite, lots of wind is needed.
- Ask participants to imagine themselves being blown about by the wind on a breezy March day.
- Select appropriate music, such as "Let's Go Fly a Kite."
- Announce that strong winds are blowing. Suggest that participants brace their bodies against the strong winds by using correct posture.
  1. Stand tall.
  2. Place the feet a little more than shoulder-width apart.
  3. Roll hips under slightly.
  4. Hold the abdomen in.
  5. Relax the shoulders.

Warm-up

1. Sway the body from side to side in a rocking motion, as though being buffeted by the wind.
2. Swing arms side to side up to shoulder height; repeat 4 times.

3. Rock from one foot to the other, lifting each foot a few inches from the floor while swinging arms from side to side. Repeat 4 times.

4. Bring arms to the front and to the back, rounding the shoulders with each move. Repeat 4 times.

5. Continue to bring arms front to back while stepping to the front, then back. Repeat 4 times.

Breathe

Prompt the group to imagine inhaling and exhaling like the whistling wind.

1. Inhale and exhale deeply. Repeat 2 times.

2. With hands at sides, inhale and raise arms out to the side and up overhead. Exhale and lower the arms back to sides.

Stretch

Arms/Shoulders: Reach up for the large cumulus clouds that pass overhead.

1. Keeping both arms up, reach up higher with one arm, then the other arm. Repeat 4 times.

2. Roll shoulders to the front and back. Repeat 4 times in each direction.

3. Pull left arm across body by grasping the left elbow with the right hand. Repeat with right arm.

Neck: Encourage the group to feel the wind blow against their cheeks, pushing their heads first in one direction, then in the other.

1. Drop arms to sides and stretch head toward the right, left, and center. Repeat 2 times.

2. Turn head and look over one shoulder, and then the other. Repeat 2 times.

Wrists/Hands

1. Roll the wrists in one direction and then the other. Repeat 2 times.

2. Wiggle the fingers; shake the hands. Repeat 2 times.

Legs

1. Bend knees slightly, then straighten them. Repeat 8 times.

2. Stretch arms high overhead and slowly roll forward toward toes. Roll up again slowly. Repeat 2 times.

DURING

Ask the group to imagine they are flying a kite that is very high in the sky. They can walk with their kite trailing behind them and they may reel it in and let it out again. Suggest that flying a kite will help give them strong arms.

1. Walk around the room with one arm extended upward (holding the kite string). To keep the arm from becoming tired, open and close the arm by moving the hand out and back to the shoulder. Change directions and begin using the other arm.

2. Bending the arms at the elbows, bring the hands in close to the chest and hold the hands one over the other, as though you are reeling in the kite.

3. Let the kite back out, circling the wrists in the opposite directions.

4. Move arms in circles by sides, moving toward the center of the room. Once in the center, lower arms and circle hands while walking backward out of the circle.

5. Put hands together and push the arms up to shoulder height and back down as if the kite is pulling the arms up. Repeat 4 times.

6. With hands still clasped, lift the arms to one side and then the other.

7. Finally, bring the kite in (reel it all the way in) while walking around the room. After all the kites are reeled in, bend over slowly and place the kite on the floor. Remember to bend the knees slightly when bending over.

8. Shake out the arms and give yourself a big hug.

AFTER

Cool down the muscles with the following movements.

1. The wind is still blowing, so sway gently from side to side, placing feet shoulder-width apart.

2. Stand tall and slowly swing arms from side to side, no higher than shoulder level.

3. Roll one shoulder, then the other, and finally both. Repeat this movement rolling first to the front and then to the back.

4. Breathe in and sweep arms out to either side. Exhale and drop the arms back to sides.

Circus of the Stars

March

> ### GOALS
> - To increase muscular strength
> - To increase flexibility
> - To explore and remember the world of the circus

MATERIALS

- Beanbags, cans of food, or other light weights
- Cassette player and cassettes

BEFORE

- Ask how many participants have watched "Circus of the Stars" on television. If they have never watched the program, explain that it is an annual show where movie stars perform circus acts. If the show is off the air or is unknown, think of this lesson as a model that can be used with some other television show or movie.

- Play appropriate music, such as "Entry of the Gladiators."

- Instruct the participants to stand like a ringmaster who must command a huge audience as well as the acts within the ring.

    1. Stand tall.
    2. Place feet shoulder-width apart.
    3. Roll hips under slightly.
    4. Tighten the abdominal muscles.
    5. Relax the shoulders.

Warm-up

Invite the group to imagine joining the circus performers as the enter the ring.

1. Form a circle (the big ring under the big top); walk around the circle, first in one direction, then the other.
2. Face the outside of the circle (the audience) and take a bow.
3. Bow again, but roll all the way down this time; roll back up slowly.

Stretch

Neck/Shoulders: Tell participants that there is so much to see that they must turn, stretch, and move in many directions.

1. Turn head to the right to see all the sights. Turn head to the left.
2. Drop the right ear toward the right shoulder, then drop the left ear toward the left shoulder. Drop head to center.
3. Roll the shoulders to the back, then roll the shoulders forward.

Arms: Suggest that participants imitate trainers as they crack the whip for the animals. Use improvised light weights during arm exercises (one 1- to 2- pound weight held in each hand). These can be small cans of food or beanbags.

1. Bring right arm in front of body, reach up, and swing down. Repeat 4 times. Alternate swinging right and left arms. Repeat each arm 4 times.
2. Circle the right arm, then the left arm in front of the body. Repeat each arm 4 times.

Legs: Direct the group to imagine the spotlight on the trapeze artist as he performs his daring act. Suggest that participants imagine what it is like to walk on the high wire.

1. Walk on tiptoes 4–6 steps.
2. Lunge forward with rear heel on floor to stretch calf; alternate legs. Repeat 4 times. Sit in a chair when finished.
3. Raise right lower leg in front of body 4 times. Raise left lower leg 4 times.
4. Walk in place lifting knees high in the air.

Feet/Ankles: Talk about circus clowns and ask participants to think of their feet as big, clumsy, clown feet.

1. Flex right foot while pointing left foot. Switch feet; repeat 4–6 times.
2. Circle the foot first to the right, then to the left. Switch feet. Repeat 4 times with each foot.

DURING

- Narrate a scene in which the participants are circus performers who are circling the ring before exiting.
- Direct participants to march in pairs around the room in tempo with the music.
  1. After one complete circle, make a half turn and march in the opposite direction around the room.

2. March a third time around the circle, crossing arms in front, separating them, and lowering them to sides.

3. Remain in a circle, open arms wide to the audience, and give yourself a big hug.

AFTER

The lesson may be concluded by asking participants if they remember going to the circus. Ask them to name their favorite circus act. To cool down, perform the following movements in circle formation.

1. Stretch arms, one after the other, toward the "tent top."

2. Face inward, take a step to the right with the right foot and slide left foot to right. Repeat with the left foot moving to the left. Repeat 4 times with each foot.

3. Shake out the right arm and then the left.

4. Shake out the right leg and then the left.

5. Breathe in deeply and exhale slowly.

Wind and Balance

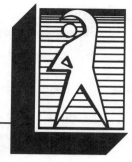

March

GOALS
• To improve balance through activity

MATERIALS

- Cassette player and cassettes

BEFORE

- Remind the group of the kinds of noises heard and the sights seen on a blustery day.
- Suggest that when the wind is strong, one must really concentrate on balance.
- Play appropriate music, such as "Oklahoma."
- Lead the group in standing up tall as a precaution from being swept away.
  1. Place feet shoulder-width apart for a strong base.
  2. Keep the knees slightly bent (soft knees).
  3. Round the pelvis under and hold in the abdomen.
  4. Relax the shoulders.

Warm-up

Encourage the group to do the warm-up exercises as if they were trees swaying in the wind.

1. Sway from side to side in a rocking motion, moving the entire body. Repeat 4 times.
2. Swing arms from side to side, up to shoulder height. Repeat 4 times.
3. Rock from one foot to the other, slightly lifting the foot. Continue swinging arms from side to side.

4. Bring arms to the front and then back, moving from the shoulder. Round the shoulders as the arms move.

5. Continue to move arms front and back. Add a step to the front, then back.

Breathe

Suggest that participants inhale and exhale like the whistling wind.

1. Inhale and exhale slowly and deeply. Repeat 2 times.

2. With hands at sides, inhale and raise arms out to the sides and up overhead. Exhale and lower the arms back to sides. Repeat 2 times.

Stretch

Arms/Shoulders: Instruct the group to reach up toward the large clouds that are racing by.

1. Move both arms overhead; stretch one arm up higher, then the other arm. Repeat 4 times.

2. Roll the shoulders to the front, gradually build up to big shoulder rolls. Repeat in the opposite direction.

3. Pull left arm across body by grasping the left elbow with the right hand. Repeat with the right arm. Repeat 2 times.

4. Take a deep breath in and open the arms wide apart.

5. Exhale and bring arms back to the center. Roll back forward and hang arms loosely in front.

Neck: Ask the group to imagine the feel of wind against their cheeks, pushing their head first in one direction, and then in the other.

1. Keep arms by sides and look first over one shoulder and then the other. Repeat 2 times.

2. Keep arms by sides and drop the head to one shoulder, and then to the other. Repeat 2 times.

Wrists/Hands

1. Rotate the wrists in one direction, then in the other. Repeat 4 times in each direction.

2. Wiggle the fingers and move them up and down as if playing a piano.

3. Shake the hands as if shaking off dishwater.

Legs

1. Bend knees and then straighten them. Repeat 8 times.

2. Stretch arms overhead and slowly roll forward toward toes. Roll up again slowly. Repeat 2 times.

DURING

Play music such as "You're Just in Love," "Surrey with the Fringe on Top," or other "Oklahoma" selections.

1. Walk between parallel lines that are spaced shoulder-width apart.
   a. Try to keep posture tall and feet between the lines.
   b. Look toward the end of the lines for better focus and direction.
   c. Repeat 3 or 4 times, or until everyone is comfortable walking down the line.
2. Stand between the lines so that one line is in front and the other is in back. Slide the feet apart and together while moving down to the end of the lines.
   a. Use arms for balance.
   b. Keep your body tall.
   c. Repeat several times.
3. Stand with feet shoulder-width apart and arms extended out to the sides.
   a. Shift weight to one foot and try to lift the other foot slightly off the floor. Switch legs.
   b. Try lifting the foot off the ground to the front, side, and rear.
   c. Maintain balance with a support (e.g., chair) and try lifting one knee up toward the front. Then move the foot back and lift it from behind.
   d. For those participants with greater flexibility, hold one foot behind the body with the opposite hand to stretch the thigh muscles (quadriceps).
4. Walk slowly across the "tightrope" (anywhere between the tape lines), practicing for the main event, and imagine having a trusty balance stick.

AFTER

1. Cool down by "walking the tightrope."
2. In the middle of the grand walk across Niagara Falls, stop and bend over to brush something off your shoe. Slowly roll up.
3. Finish by taking a bow, with hat in hand (of course).

SAFETY PRECAUTIONS

Suggest that participants hold the back of a chair for balance while shifting weight from one foot to the other.

Happy Times

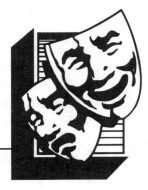

March

MATERIALS
- Chalkboard or large piece of paper
- Chalk or something else with which to write

BEFORE
1. Ask participants to recall a happy time in their lives.
2. On the chalkboard or on a large piece of paper, make a list of these events (e.g., getting a puppy or a toy as a child, playing ball with a sibling, getting engaged or married).

DURING
1. Form the participants into small groups of about three people.
2. Ask the group to select 1 or 2 episodes from the above list to act out in a skit. Have them plan and practice their skits.
3. Ask participants to rehearse their skits for the rest of the group.
4. After each skit, lead the group in commenting on how the actors conveyed different actions and ideas to the audience.
5. Ask each participant how they felt about the character they portrayed and what memories the exercise brought to mind.

AFTER
With the group's help, make a list of the small things everyone can do the rest of the day to bring more happiness to the world.

Imagination

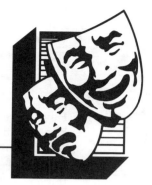

March

BEFORE

1. Introduce the topic of remembering kites through imagination.

2. Let each person find a partner and instruct them to sit facing each other.

3. Direct one person to move and the other to mirror those movements. Suggest that in addition to the movements the participants create, they make the following movements, too: blow like a strong March wind, hiss like lightning, clap like thunder, and fall like gentle rain.

4. Tell the pairs to switch roles. The next set of movements could include: blowing like a gentle breeze, acting like bird caught in a wind storm, and rushing like a river.

DURING

1. Tell the groups to remain in pairs.

2. Ask one person in each pair to pretend to be a kite and the other to pretend to fly the kite. Explain that while they are playing on a sunny, warm, March day, the clouds begin rolling in and it becomes windy. As time passes, it becomes very windy and begins to drizzle. Finally, the weather becomes sunny and warm again.

3. Ask each pair to demonstrate how they would react due to the change in weather.

4. Let the pairs switch roles.

5. Ask everyone to come back together and form a circle.

6. Begin a group pantomime by asking all of the participants to pantomime their answers to such questions as: How did it feel to be a kite on a stormy, windy day? The string breaks and you are free, what happens and how do you feel? What does the flyer do and how does the kite flyer feel when the string breaks?

AFTER

1. Have a group discussion on freedom and limitations. Ask if they think the kite goes higher when it is free or when it is restrained on a string. Ask the participants if there is any parallel to that in life, as they have seen it.

2. Inquire if people "go higher" when they have responsibilities that restrain them or when they are totally free.

3. The leader or participants may share stories of freedom and restraint when they were raising children or when they were young.

4. A balloon could be inflated and let go, flapping wildly with its air rushing out.

5. Ask participants if, at this time of their lives, they seem to be on a string or free, and if there any ways they could change these feelings.

Movement and Imagination

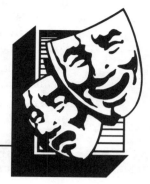

March

MATERIALS

- Weather map from the newspaper (optional)
- Cassette player and cassette of the sounds of wind (optional)

BEFORE

1. Form the group into a circle.
2. Invite the group to pantomime blowing up an imaginary balloon, letting the air out, and passing the imaginary balloon to the person to their left.
3. Play a tape with wind sounds or assign certain group members to make wind noises.
4. Direct the group to pantomime holding a balloon. Tell the group that as they hear the wind blowing it will become harder to control the balloon.
5. Slowly increase the intensity of the wind sounds. Explain that the balloon is steadily becoming larger and that the wind is blowing hard. All the participants must hold on to the balloon in order to maintain control. Because the balloon is so large it will eventually float away.

DURING

1. Divide the group into pairs. Pair up individuals with mental disabilities with individuals without mental disabilities if possible. This activity requires a lot of space, so instruct participants to leave plenty of space between them.

2. Instruct each pair to pretend to have a pole between them that is about 20 feet tall. The pole is held only by their stomachs. They must keep the pole in the middle of their bodies. The pairs can move backward and forward, side to side, but they cannot drop the pole. They can stretch their body, raise their arms above their head, and place their feet out to the sides while keeping the pole between them.

3. Suggest that they grab the pole and plant one end of it in the ground so that it can become a flagpole.

4. Give each pair an imaginary package that contains a 6-foot American flag to be run up their pole. Tell the pairs to keep the flag from touching the ground.

5. After the flag is at the top of the pole, tell the pairs that they must hold it steady because there is a breeze. Explain that there is a sudden clap of thunder in the distance and that the wind begins to blow stronger and stronger. The pole sways and the flag whips wildly. Have participants enact sounds and actions of the flag flapping and the wind blowing.

6. Each pair must lower the flag, lay down the pole, and fold the flag during the wind storm. Allow adequate time for the participants to fold their imaginary flags and stack the imaginary flagpoles in the corner.

AFTER

1. During a group discussion, ask about how the pairs worked together in maintaining balance of the pole and in folding the flag.

2. Using a weather map from the newspaper, discuss where the wind comes from and differences in air pressure, fronts, highs, and lows.

3. Talk with the group about how terminology about the wind has been used to convey emotions; for example, whether they have ever been in a dither, on cloud nine, or raced around like a tornado.

Creating Mobiles

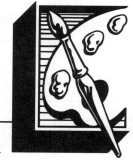

March

GOALS

- To create mobiles
- To observe the effects of wind
- To explore wind as a theme in art

MATERIALS

- Heavy gauge wire, tree branches, or dowel sticks can be used as armature depending on the type of mobile
- Clear fishing line (excellent for attaching shapes and forms to the armature)
- Natural objects such as tree limbs, pine cones, shells with holes in them, and twigs
- Buttons, old jewelry, kitchen utensils, discarded tools, plastic flowers—absolutely anything with an interesting shape or color can take on a new identity when it becomes a part of the mobile
- Colored tag board or poster board
- Scissors
- Glue
- Wind chime or completed mobile
- Pictures or photographs of John Constable's paintings of clouds or of Alexander Calder's mobiles. Books about these two artists' work can be found at most local libraries.

BEFORE

1. Discuss characteristics of spring weather with the group. Focus on the wind as a powerful element of nature. Ask how wind sounds, feels, and looks. What is the function of wind and how does it relate to their lives?

---

2. Present visuals that show the effects of windy weather (trees blowing, kites soaring, people holding onto hats, aftermath of tornadoes, sailing ships).

3. Ask participants to share "wind experiences."

4. Discuss wind as a theme in art. If possible, bring in an example of a recording, painting, or sculpture that shows the effects of wind.

5. Have a wind chime or mobile to present to the group. Let participants observe how movement and balance are determined by the shape and weight of objects. Help them see that in a mobile, movement and space, as well as the objects themselves, become a part of the sculpture.

DURING

1. Distribute materials for creating mobiles. Natural objects can be made into attractive wind sculptures. Use an interesting tree branch as an anchor for suspending pine cones, shells, and twigs.

2. Participants may enjoy going outside the facility to look for things they can incorporate into their sculpture. Clear fishing line is excellent for attaching the objects they find.

3. Participants may want to play a larger role in designing their mobiles. Dowel sticks or heavy wire make an excellent armature, and colored poster board or tag board offers them a variety of choices.

4. Ask questions to promote aesthetic thinking: Do you want shapes in your mobile to represent something realistic or would you prefer them to be abstract? Would you like your mobile to be a mixture of nature and man-made objects? Do you want a variety of colors in your mobile or will you choose to have one dominant color? How will you balance the weight of objects that you use?

5. After participants choose objects or create shapes for their mobiles, have them attach them to the armature with the fishing twine. Working with a partner is helpful at this stage. One person can help another to balance the weight of objects. One partner can hold up the mobile while the other watches how objects move in space.

AFTER

1. Have participants look at each other's mobiles before they are hung. Discuss each individual's choice of shapes and colors and prompt a dialogue within the group. "Why did you choose these specific objects? How did you solve the problem of balance as you designed your sculpture?"

2. Hang the mobiles and observe the effect of movement and space on the sculptures. Find words to describe how forms move in the wind (slowly, smoothly, freely).

3. Encourage participants to think of themselves as forms in space. Can they move like their mobiles? How important is personal space? Is the space environment at the facility comfortable? Discuss the importance of having enough emotional and personal space.

ADAPTATION

Art materials can provide exciting stimulation to persons with visual impairment. Participants can assist in gathering art media such as the following:

- Textured papers (e.g., sandpaper of varying degrees of coarseness)
- Boldly patterned papers, wallpaper, and wrapping paper
- Thick yarn or cord with which to hang the shapes
- Materials that create sound when swaying in the breeze and touching other objects
- Large shapes in very bold colors

Cloud Paintings

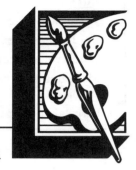

March

GOALS
- To create murals using oil pastel/resist technique
- To focus on the sense of sight by observing colors and shapes of clouds
- To share memories of outdoor experiences
- To experiment with mixing colors

MATERIALS
- Photographs, slides, and other images of clouds and sky
- Oil pastels (crayons will do if applied heavily)
- Block tempera paints
- Brushes
- Water
- Two or three long pieces of white mural paper
- Books with illustrations of the work of Georgia O'Keefe and John Constable (optional), which can be found at local libraries

BEFORE
1. Ask the group to look out the window or go outdoors to look at the sky.
2. If it is a day with distant clouds, ask participants to use their imaginations and look for images in cloud shapes. Encourage the group to look at the sky at different times of day.
3. Present images of the sky. Encourage close observation by asking questions such as: What colors do you see in the sky? Describe colors that are typical of morning, midday, and late afternoon. What is your favorite time of day? What colors would you find in the sky then?
4. Discuss the shape and color of clouds in various pictures.

DURING

1. Divide participants into two or three groups. Each group will create a large painting of the sky, deciding first what time of day they want to portray.

2. Using oil pastels (or heavy application of crayons) to create cloud shapes, have participants layer colors and experiment with blending the oil pastels (e.g., white and red create pink, yellow and blue create green). The group may choose to incorporate other shapes in their sky mural—birds, planes, hot air balloons, and so forth.

3. After oil pastel work is complete, pass out block tempera paint. Using a good bit of water on the brush, apply paint over cloud shapes and fill in the background of sky. The tempera paint will not cover up the oil pastels, but will color the background and leave a lovely textured effect on clouds.

AFTER

1. Look at the murals while they are drying. Discuss colors, shapes of clouds, and time of day. Prompt dialogue about the process of creating the mural. Ask what the participants discovered about color mixing. Point out an especially beautiful color and ask the participant how he or she made it.

2. Share memories of times spent outdoors when the sky was very colorful.

3. Ask the group if they can see the sunrise or sunset from their homes or rooms.

4. Urge the group to be aware of the sky and to look for any of the colors they mixed for the mural.

5. Hang sky murals on the walls at the facility for all to enjoy.

Japanese Fish Kites

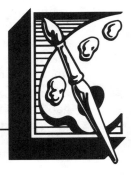

March

GOALS

- To reminisce about experiences with kites
- To become familiar with the art of Japanese kite making
- To explore printing as a decorative technique
- To create decorative fish kites

MATERIALS

- Pictures of fish
- Large white sheets of paper (18" × 24") folded in half lengthwise
- Scissors
- Pencils and markers
- Staplers
- Cellophane tape
- Tempera paint and small sponges
- Small bowls
- Objects for printing (corks, erasers, paper clips, small rectangles of corrugated cardboard, shells, etc.)
- Thin wire or balsa wood

BEFORE

1. Announce that March is traditionally the month for flying kites. Ask the participants to reminisce about experiences they have had in the past with kites. Ask anyone in the group who has made a kite to share his or her experience in kite making and flying.

2. Explain that in Japan kite making is an art. Entire villages work together to create kites for yearly competitions. One of the most popular types of kites in Japan is the fish kite, which works something like a windsock. It is in the shape of a fish with its mouth open. Wind fills the body of the fish and causes the kite to lift and fly. These kites can be very beautiful, patterned with many shapes and colors, with streamers or ribbons hanging from the tail of the fish.

3. After telling the group some of the history of kite making, reveal that they are going to create decorative fish kites using an object-printing technique.

DURING

1. Have two or three visuals of fish for the group to look at. Point out the overall shape of the body and look carefully at the shapes and patterns created by fins, scales, and so forth.

2. Demonstrate how to draw a simple fish shape. Practice on a piece of newsprint, then draw the fish on a folded sheet of white paper. One side of the fish must be against the fold of the paper, and the mouth opening must be fairly large.

3. After participants have outlined the fish with pencil on their paper, they are ready to add details. Have the group lightly sketch in the face of their fish with a pencil, then add fins, tail, and any other major shapes they wish to include.

4. Go over the pencil lines with colored markers.

5. Cut out the body of the fish, being careful not to cut into the fold of the paper.

6. Fold the mouth of the fish back to the outside about 1" to create a sleeve through which to put a piece of balsa.

7. Hand out containers with paint-soaked sponges. (These should be prepared ahead of time by diluting tempera paint and pouring it over small squares of sponges in plastic bowls. This creates a type of stamp pad.)

8. Hand out objects for printing. Have the participants choose one or two objects and then encourage them to create interesting patterns on the body of their fish kite. They may wish to use markers first, drawing scales on the body and then adding more decorative shapes by printing on top. This is the time for the group to be creative, have fun, and to find solutions that are pleasing to them.

AFTER

1. When the fish kites are dry, have the group complete them by stapling together the open side of fish body, attaching colored ribbons to the tail of the kite, and threading a piece of thin wire or balsa wood through the sleeve of paper around its mouth.

2. Kites can be hung around the facility providing a colorful visual appropriate to "windy," spring kite weather.

3. Perhaps some participants have grandchildren or young friends with which they would like to share their kite.

ADAPTATION

The fish pattern may pose difficulty for participants who cannot visualize the eventual three-dimensional shape. They may require extra guidance or a friend to help them during this or any other phase that proves too difficult. The printing, however, with found objects should be exciting for all.

Patterns of the Body

March

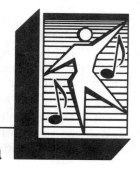

GOALS

- To explore making circles with the body—with isolated body parts, with the whole body, and together with others
- To learn to recognize abstract shapes in unusual places
- To consider the roles cycles play in life
- To create a "massage circle"

MATERIALS

- Pictures of circular things, such as umbrellas, the solar system, atoms, ripples in water, cakes, wheels, rings, records on turntables, coiled snakes, bowls or plates, or open mouths

BEFORE

Ask participants what all the pictures have in common. Then ask them to look around the room and see what kinds of circles they can find.

DURING

1. Divide the participants into groups of approximately five. Have them stand in circles facing inward.

2. Tell everyone to begin by making a circle with one finger. Then ask them to circle the big toe of the opposite foot. Advise participants to hold onto the back of a chair for balance. Next, tell them to circle the wrist, moving the whole hand, and then the opposite ankle. Proceed to the lower arm from the elbow, then the lower leg from the knee. Tell participants to circle one shoulder, both forward and back, and then circle the thigh of the opposite leg. Repeat, using the opposite shoulder and thigh. Ask them to let the head

roll in a circle, being careful not to let it drop too far back. Make sure it circles at least once to each side. Tell them to try making circles with just the ribs (this is a hard one). Then suggest making circles with the hips. The hips and ribs can circle both side to side, front to back, and up and down.

3. Instead of using only one body part at a time, tell participants to put them all together. Use the whole arm or circle the whole upper body. There is no right or wrong way to move. Encourage everyone to experiment; if someone is doing something interesting, let the group see it. Tell people to "borrow" moves from each other if they see something they like, but to keep exploring. There are many different ways to make circles with the body.

4. Direct participants to begin circling in place. Let the circles become steps so that participants are walking in individual circles. Let these circles "grow" until each group is walking in a small circle together. Let this circle "grow" until everyone is walking together in a big circle. Participants should feel free to continue making circular movements with their bodies as they walk in these circles. Be careful that participants do not become dizzy and fall from enthusiastic circling.

5. Ask everyone to stop walking, face the center of the big circle, and come in so that they are shoulder to shoulder.

6. Tell participants to turn in the same direction so that they are all facing someone's back. Direct participants to put their hands on the shoulders of the person in front of them and to imagine that they are typing on a typewriter in slow motion. This should feel really good on the participants' shoulders. Tell everyone to ask the person in front of them how much pressure they want on their shoulders. People usually want more than other people think they do. Encourage people not to be afraid to go ahead and press hard. Keep this movement going for a while.

7. Ask everyone to stop "typing" and stroke briskly from the neck to shoulder three times, as if they were wiping off the person's shoulders.

8. Tell participants to rub their hands together, as if they were warming them, then tell them to make a ball with their hands that holds all of the tension they took out of that person's shoulders. Count to three and have everyone throw that tension away outside the circle together.

AFTER

Instruct everyone to sit in a circle to share experiences. Discuss life's circular patterns. There are many cycles in nature (water cycles, seasons, plant life) and some people find that there are cycles in human life as well. How do people feel about this idea? Has history repeated itself in people's lives? What cycles and circles do people see in the world?

Beginning with Breath

March

GOALS
• To gain an increased awareness of breath • To explore breath's relationship to movement

BEFORE

1. Introduce the idea of breath as the "wind" in the body. Tell the group that they will be working with breath in this activity. Instruct participants to listen to their own bodies and not to force a pattern of breathing that is uncomfortable. As they work with different types of breathing, they should allow themselves to rest and breathe normally whenever they feel the need. Sometimes breathing, especially deeply, quickly, or forcefully, can make people feel lightheaded or unsteady. Encourage participants to pay attention to how they are feeling. As the leader, watch for people who are doing too much.

2. Begin by having participants sit in a circle with their eyes closed.

3. In a slow, gentle voice, direct them to sit quietly until they notice the pattern of their breathing. Advise them not to try to breathe any special way, but to breathe naturally.

4. Direct participants to breathe a little more deeply and slowly. Tell them to breathe in through the nose and breathe out through the mouth, letting the jaw slacken. Remind them not to force the breathing, but to do what is comfortable and relaxing for them.

DURING

1. While seated, direct participants to take the motion of the breath into their bodies. As they breathe in, have them lift their shoulders up to their ears.

As they breathe out, have them release their shoulders. (If they wish, they may open their eyes at this point. If you sense that being visible to others is inhibiting people, help them adjust their chairs so that they are facing away from the group.)

2. As they breathe in, tell them to lift up an arm. As they breathe out, tell them to drop that arm. As they breathe in, have them lift their upper bodies. As they breathe out have them slacken their bodies.

3. Encourage everyone to let the movement come from the breath. If they are having trouble with this, demonstrate a few movements for them.

4. Ask those who can to stand up.

5. Direct everyone to face different directions so that they can concentrate on how the movement feels to them and not how it looks to someone else.

6. Allow the group to experiment with more breath movements in the same even in-and-out rhythm. Let them see how many parts of their bodies they can involve. If they wish, they may hold the backs of chairs for balance. Remind them once more to stop and breathe normally if they feel uncomfortable or lightheaded. If the group is getting bogged down doing the same kinds of movements, here are some suggestions:

   Rise up as you breathe in, drop or collapse as you breathe out.

   Open up the body as you breathe in, close up the body as you breathe out.

   Close up the body as you breathe in, open up the body as you breathe out.

   Turn to the right as you breathe in, to the left as you breathe out.

7. Encourage them to travel throughout the room while making the breathing movements.

8. Ask the group to experiment with different breath rhythms. They may choose to breathe in and out quickly, to breathe in slowly and breathe out quickly, or the reverse. Have them mix these different rhythms, always moving along with their breath.

9. After they have worked with this for about 5 minutes, have the group split in half with each half watching the other.

AFTER

Concentration on breath can be very relaxing. Ask the group if they felt relaxed, centered, or focused when they were involved in the breath exercises. If so, suggest that they experiment this week with taking 15 minutes, perhaps in the very beginning of the day, to concentrate on breathing. Suggest that this activity will make them more focused and comfortable throughout the day.

Note

Watch for people who are overexerting or breathing strangely. Remind participants that if they feel uncomfortable or lightheaded at any time during the lesson, they should stop and breathe normally.

Storm of Sound and Motion

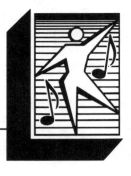

March

GOALS

- To enjoy a collaborative creative experience
- To explore the same phenomenon—a thunderstorm—through two expressive forms: sound and movement

MATERIALS

- Percussion instruments, musical instruments, or noisemakers to make a thunderstorm
- Cassette player
- Recordings of rain and thunder (these are available at many record stores and libraries)

BEFORE

1. Ask the group to talk about thunderstorms they remember. Ask if anyone has any good stories to tell about especially big storms. What are the elements of a thunderstorm? Some answers might be: gathering clouds; flashes of lightning; peals of thunder; a sudden downpour; light, misty rain; the smell of wet earth; wind; dripping eaves; overflowing gutters; umbrellas; puddles; wet shoes and clothes; hearing the rain come down harder and faster; the sound of rain on the roof or on an awning; raindrops running down a window; the sound of windshield wipers; or cars spraying pedestrians.

2. Divide the group in half. One half will be the sounds of the storm and the other half will be the storm in movement.

3. Let the sound group decide what part of the storm they want to play: rain, thunder, lightning, wind, or something else. Let them choose the instru-

ments that are best for their roles. Participants can use instruments, make sounds with their voices, or invent an instrument from something in the room. Someone might even want to flick the lights on and off for lightning.

4. As the "orchestra" is getting itself together, the movers can start to experiment with different movements. They can decide to choose one element of the storm and stay with that (e.g., clouds, rain, wind) or they can shift from one element to another as the spirit moves them.

DURING

1. Let the storm begin. Have the orchestra sit together with their instruments on one side of the room facing the movers and let them begin to play.

2. Movers can choose to enter, exit, move, freeze, interact with each other, or go solo. Movers might want to focus on one instrument and the sound it makes, or choose not to connect their movement with any sound at all.

3. After about 5 minutes, let the groups switch. A variation would be to use a call and respond pattern with the orchestra making storm sounds and then the movers responding to the sounds in silence.

AFTER

1. Play some gentle rain sounds on a cassette player and have people come together in a circle to cool down.

2. Have the group follow the slow, easy movements of one person—like group mirroring.

3. As the leader, you might want to begin leading and then pass the leadership on to someone else.

ADAPTATION

It may not be appropriate to ask persons with behavior disorders to move like a violent storm or make loud noises. If this is true of some participants, tame the storm to a light shower and emphasize other nonviolent qualities of rain.

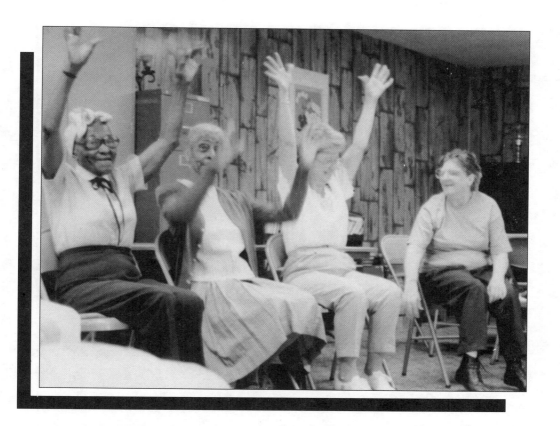

April

Themes:

Flowers
Colors
Humor
Playfulness
Amusement
Spontaneity
Social interaction

Spring Cleaning

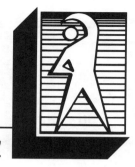

April

GOALS

- To increase cardiorespiratory endurance through aerobic dance
- To improve self-concept through improved movement proficiency

---

MATERIALS

- Cassette player and cassettes

BEFORE

- Offer a few suggestions of spring cleaning warm-up activities. Encourage participants to add other activities.
- Select music such as "Here You Come Again" by Dolly Parton.
- Direct participants to use correct posture.
    1. Stand or sit up tall.
    2. Press lower back into chair; if standing, roll hips (pelvis) slightly under.
    3. Tighten the abdomen.

Warm-up

Ask participants to "clean house." Repeat each activity 8 times.

1. Open up the drapes—push arms out to sides and reach out.
2. Reach up and clean the windows—circle hands around and reach up. (Make sure you get the corners.)
3. Open the window—stretch arms up.
4. Wash clothes—bend and straighten arms, moving hands in and out in front of the body.

---

5. Hang clothes on the line—squat down and pick up an imaginary article of clothing and pin it on the line.

Breathe

Urge the participants to take in fresh, spring air with every breath.

1. Open the window for fresh air—push arms up, then bring them down.
2. Inhale and exhale several times slowly and deeply.
3. Close the window—reach up, then bring arms down.

Stretch

Neck: Roll the neck to the right, center, and left. Repeat 6–8 times.

Shoulders

1. Roll the shoulders to the front and back. Repeat 6 times in each direction.
2. Stretch the shoulders by giving yourself a hug; then pull the right arm across the chest by holding the right elbow with the left hand; release and switch arms.

Arms: Circle arms with the arms straight out to the sides. Make small circles and increase the circle to the maximum size. Return to starting position. Repeat 6–8 times.

Back: Touch toes by rolling the back down with arms overhead. If standing, keep knees slightly bent (to protect the lower back).

Legs

1. Extend legs out in front of the body while seated to stretch the hamstrings. Extend one leg and then the other.
2. Stretch the legs while seated by pulling one knee in toward the chest; drop leg and switch.

DURING

Begin with arm exercises similar to those practiced during the warm-up, but play music with a faster tempo, such as "You Are My Sunshine."

1. Open up the drapes—push arms out to sides; reach out, then bring arms in. Repeat 6–8 times.
2. Reach up and clean the windows alternating one arm and then the other; circle hands around while reaching up.
3. Open the windows—stretch arms up and down, up and down.
4. Wash clothes—bend and straighten arms, moving hands in and out in front of the body.
5. Hang clothes on the line—bend over and pick up an imaginary article of clothing and pin it on the line.

Dance #1

Play upbeat music, such as "Rock Around the Clock." Ask everyone to stand in a circle and follow these steps:

1. Move right foot out to the side 2 times.
2. Move left foot out to the side 2 times.
3. Step up on the right foot, bring left foot together with right foot.
4. Step back on the right foot, move left foot next to right foot.
5. Walk forward 3 steps, then bring feet together. Repeat 1 time.

Assess heart rate and rate of perceived exertion after the dance. (Charts to measure these rates can be found in the Fitness section of Chapter 3.) Start over with step 1 and repeat until music ends.

Dance #2

This dance is similar to Dance #1, but it adds arm movements. Play music, such as "Sun in the Morning" and follow these steps:

1. Move right foot out to the side and back in 4 times. Swing arms out and in with foot.
2. Walk forward 6 steps.
3. Stop, bring feet together, and clap twice with the music.
4. Move left foot out to the side and back in 4 times. Swing arms out and in with the foot.
5. Walk forward 6 steps.
6. Stop, bring feet together, and clap twice.

Assess heart rate and rate of perceived exertion after the dance. Start over with step 1 and repeat until music ends. Stress arm movement.

AFTER

Ask participants to form a circle and face the center.

1. Roll shoulders back, one at a time, slowly.
2. Repeat slow shoulder rolls to the front.
3. Interlace fingers and push palms of hands out in front of body.
4. Reach up overhead and stretch arms out to the sides and back down.
5. Give yourself a hug.

Finish the session by assessing recovery heart rate and rate of perceived exertion.

Spring Chickens

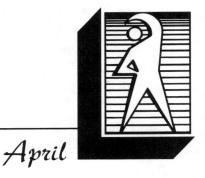

April

GOALS

- To become more aware of good posture by focusing on body alignment
- To continue to improve cardiorespiratory endurance through walking

BEFORE

Announce that spring has finally arrived and that there is excitement in the air. Urge participants to think about the new possibilities that spring brings. List their ideas on a chalkboard. Direct participants to use correct posture.

1. Stand tall or sit up straight; be proud.
2. Round the pelvis under and hold in the stomach muscles.
3. Relax the shoulders.

Warm-up

1. Reach up to the sky and open arms to greet the fresh day.
2. Move arms out to the sides and lower them slowly.
3. Reach arms up once more and roll down to see the flowers starting to bloom.
4. Walk briskly in place to the beat of lively music.

Breathe

1. Inhale and exhale slowly several times—in through the nose and out through the mouth.
2. Lift the arms up overhead and slowly bend over to touch toes.

Stretch

Neck: Turn head from side to side and greet your neighbor with a smile. Hold each position 10–15 seconds.

Shoulders

1. Roll shoulders to the front 6–8 times and back 6–8 times.
2. Give yourself a hug; then hold the right arm across the body by holding the left elbow; switch arms.

Arms: Alternately reach arms up, one arm higher than the other each time.

Back: Roll over with arms overhead and try to touch toes. If standing, keep knees slightly bent. Repeat 6–8 times.

Upper torso and legs: Bend forward from the hips, keeping legs straight and leading with the chin. Raise arms as high behind the back as possible, keeping elbows straight and palms together. Hold 10–15 seconds.

Calves: Stand 2–3 feet away from the wall with hands placed on the wall at eye level. Keep heels on floor while continuing to lean forward. Hold 10–15 seconds.

DURING

Lead the group on a walk outside. Ask them to concentrate on tall posture and to carefully swing their arms. After walking for about 5 minutes, stop and ask participants to assess their pulse rate. Instruct them to think about how hard they are walking. Continue walking.

AFTER

1. Walk back into the building and make a circle.
2. Stretch the arms overhead and then relax them by the sides.
3. Sit in a chair and do 4–5 ankle circles with each foot.

SAFETY PRECAUTIONS

Advise the group to keep knees bent when attempting to touch their toes to avoid undue stress on the knees and back.

Showers, Flowers, and Rainbows

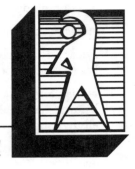

April

GOALS

- To increase range of movement through flexibility exercises
- To increase aerobic fitness through walking

BEFORE

Begin session by asking participants to think about the last week in April and the things that are associated with it, such as showers, thunderstorms, rainbows, flowers, and so forth.

Warm-up

Tell the group that there is something about this time of year that makes people aware of the positive aspects of nature. Ask what kind of weather April means for them.

1. Walk in place, swinging arms and crossing arms in front of body, then out to the sides. Repeat 8 times.
2. Walk 4 steps with feet side by side, 4 steps with feet shoulder-width apart, then 4 steps with feet side by side again.
3. Standing in a stationary position, swing arms up and toward ceiling, then down toward floor. Inhale as arms swing up, exhale as arms swing down. Repeat 8 times.

Stretch

Neck: Suggest that participants pretend to look at flowers as they turn their necks.

1. Turn neck to the left, center, and right. Hold each position for 10 seconds.
2. Repeat in each direction 6–8 times.

Arms/Shoulders:　Suggest that participants imagine clouds forming overhead.

1.   Alternately extend right and left arms overhead as if trying to touch the clouds. Repeat 8 times.

2.   Shrug shoulders simultaneously as if reacting to the rain. Alternately shrug and relax 8 times.

3.   Extend arms out to the sides at shoulder level with palms downward. Rotate both arms so palms are facing up. Repeat rotations 8 times.

Wrists/Hands:　Encourage participants to mimic the soft falling of spring rain with their fingers.

1.   Bend arms and point hands upward while slowly wiggling and stretching the fingers.

2.   With arms still bent, turn wrists as if twirling the handle of an umbrella. Repeat with each hand 8 times.

Sides:　Describe a day when the winds are getting stronger and umbrellas are becoming difficult to keep upright.

1.   Stand with feet shoulder-width apart.

2.   Let one arm hang to the side. Extend the other arm up over the head (as if holding an umbrella).

3.   Bend slowly toward the side with the arm hanging down and stretch as far as is comfortable.

4.   Return to an upright position.

5.   Repeat, stretching to the opposite side.

6.   Repeat stretches 8 times to each side.

Legs:　Describe an afternoon when a heavy rain has stopped and a rainbow is forming in the sky.

1.   Holding the back of a chair if necessary, shift weight forward and stand on tiptoes. Hold for 10 seconds. Lower feet and repeat 6–8 times.

2.   Holding the back of a chair, extend the right leg backward and hold for 10 seconds. Repeat with the left leg. Alternate 6–8 times.

3.   Flex and extend each foot 8–10 times.

DURING

Describe how pleasant it is after a spring rain. Tell participants to smell the freshness of the air and flowers, see the bright shiny leaves and the rainbow, and feel the brightness of the sun.

Lead participants in an outdoor walk. Walk approximately ¼–½ mile. Be sure participants check their pulse rates at the completion of the walk.

AFTER

Ask participants to start thinking about the month of May and the activities and thoughts that they associate with that month.

1.   Walk slowly around the room, in place or forward and back.

2. Breath in and out slowly.
3. Swing both arms, alternating to left and right.

SAFETY PRECAUTIONS

Stress the importance of holding the back of a chair for support when on tiptoes or when one foot is off the floor.

Humor and Fun

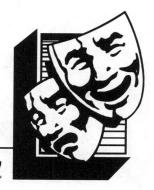

GOALS
• To laugh
• To make others laugh

BEFORE

1. Introduce the activity by talking about humor and comedy in drama.

2. Ask each person if he or she has heard a good joke recently. Ask those who know a joke to tell it.

3. Begin a group discussion by asking each of the participants such questions as: What is humor? What are types of humor? Is laughter really the best medicine? What makes you laugh?

DURING

1. Invite the group to participate in a game called "Make me laugh!"

2. Place three chairs together for the stage. Ask the participants to move their chairs in a semicircle around the other three.

3. Explain that the purpose of the game is for the audience to try to make the three people on stage laugh. Tell the audience that they may make faces, move about, dance, make noises, laugh out loud in all sorts of ways, and so forth. If any of the three people on stage laughs, he or she must join the audience.

4. Ask for volunteers to sit in the chairs on the stage. Make sure that everyone in the audience gets a chance to be on the "Can't-Make-Me-Laugh" panel.

AFTER

1. Begin a group discussion by asking each of the participants which actions made him or her laugh the hardest and why.

2. Determine through discussion if some participants have a special gift for making people laugh. Perhaps the group can figure out how they do this or the people can tell what their secret is to making people laugh.

3. Ask again if anyone has a joke to share with the group.

ADAPTATION

For individuals with mental retardation or dementia who cannot remember a funny story or joke, the leader can help them to participate by bringing newspaper cartoons for them to discuss. They can explain who is depicted doing what actions. Another way is to show a video and to stop it after funny episodes and then have the individuals tell you about the funny episode that occurred.

Laughter

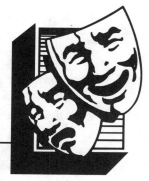

April

GOALS

- To relax through laughter
- To make clown movements
- To remember great clowns
- To create a clown skit

MATERIALS

- VCR and a rented funny video
- Video camera to record the participants laughing (optional)
- Chalkboard or large piece of paper
- Chalk or something else with which to write

BEFORE

Introduce the topic of laughter and talk about how it is known as the "best medicine." Begin a group discussion on how laughter helps people stay healthy. Participants can do a poll to verify the truth of this—they can name people they know who laugh a lot and try to remember whether these people seem healthier than most people.

DURING

1. Clowns have always been a source of laughter. Ask the group to name some famous clowns and comedians, such as the Marx Brothers, Lucille Ball, W.C. Fields, Charlie Chaplin, the Three Stooges, Gilda Radner, Elaine Boozler, Bill Cosby, and Buster Keaton. Their names can be written on a chalkboard.

2. Lead the group in role-playing clown movements, such as a big smile, eye winks, shoulder shrugs, eye rolling, arm swings, and exaggerated leg movements.

3. Have the group experiment with different kinds of laughs: high quick tittering laughs, belly laughs, muffled hidden laughs, laughs through our noses with our mouths closed, laughs with our mouths wide open, mischievous laughs, and laughs that shake our whole body and double us over. The group can give names to the several kinds of laughter and list them on a chalkboard.

4. Divide the participants into groups of three or four.

5. Have each group put on a laughing act for the rest of the group to see how much the audience will laugh for each act. As a part of their laughing act, the members can share their favorite comedy scenes or enact funny situations.

AFTER

Rent a funny video to watch as a group. Urge the participants to practice an assortment of new ways of laughing as they watch the video. If one joke is particularly funny, help them to remember it and to share it with others throughout the day.

April Showers and Spring Flowers

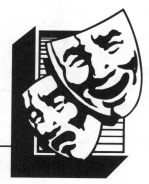

April

MATERIALS

- Chalkboard and chalk

BEFORE

1. Introduce the topic of April showers and spring flowers. This is a good activity for a rainy day.

2. Ask the participants to tell about their circumstances during the worst rain and the most pleasant rain they have ever experienced. Record the responses of the participants on a chalkboard.

3. Begin a discussion about flowers. Tell the group that flowers bloom every spring. Ask such questions as: What kinds of flowers bloom first? Which ones and which colors are your favorite?

4. To warm up the group for telling stories about themselves and flowers, the leader should first tell a story about when he or she received, gave, picked, or grew a flower.

5. Ask participants in the group to make up a story or tell the group a story that involves a flower.

DURING

1. To do a "rainy" skit, divide the group into pairs.

2. Have each group act out different kinds of rains or a combination of rains. Some skits might be about a gentle rain, a thunderstorm, an icy rain, or the

end of a rain when the sun comes out. During the rain, the actors may pretend that they are falling in love with each other in the rain or having a fight while carrying home paper bags of groceries that burst from wetness.

3. Another exercise is to have participants pretend that they are a flower seed or bulb of a special type; for example, a seed that grows to be a Manhattan taxi driver, a princess, or a muscle man. Encourage participants to think of their own types of flowers or bulbs.

4. Discuss how they might break through the ground and bloom.

5. Form the group into a semicircle and give everyone a few chances to perform. Change the weather conditions during each scene.

AFTER

Suggest that members of the group create a garden or grow some bulbs either at the facility or at home. The flowers can then be given the names of characters that the participants played in the drama session and each pot can be individually labeled.

ADAPTATION

Persons with good knowledge of weather conditions and good memories can add scientific information, such as typical weather patterns and the average number of inches of rain per year. Folk methods of weather forecasting can be discussed; for example, "red sky at night, sailor's delight; red sky in the morning, sailor's warning." The leader can help by bringing in the daily newspaper's weather page to spur the discussion. Participants can tell how the weather differs in various regions of the country where they have lived and tell of floods and droughts they remember. Whenever the leader suspects that gifted individuals are not challenged by the content, take this kind of intellectual, scientific approach in order to add an intellectually challenging dimension to the activity. Also, it is not necessary that the leader knows the answers, it is only necessary that the leader has the capacity to lead the participants in thinking about a topic.

Sculpting Memories in Clay

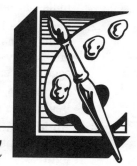

April

GOALS

- To create a sculpture from clay to illustrate a spring experience
- To reminisce about experiences of birth and renewal in spring
- To discuss the value of caring and nurturing for others

MATERIALS

- Images of growth, renewal, or nurturing (e.g., illustrations of paintings by Mary Cassatt, who captures moments of caring and nurturing between mother and child)
- Magazine pictures of adults and children, animals, gardens, or spring scenes
- Clay (1 pound per person)
- Burlap squares or newspapers
- Toothpicks
- Plastic forks
- Small containers for water

BEFORE

1. Discuss memories of spring that involve birth and renewal, such as planting a garden and watching seed sprout and grow. Other spring memories may include observing trees bud and develop leaves, enjoying the beauty of nature as colorful flowers appear, or noticing newborn animals in fields.

2. Ask the group questions about birth and renewal: Who has cared for a newborn creature, perhaps a family pet? How have you given expression to those kinds of nurturing feelings in your adult life? What was it like raising children, grandchildren, or pets? What are some ways you show caring and nurturing for others?

DURING

1. View some images that illustrate growth, renewal, or nurturing. These could include magazine photographs of adults and children, young animals, gardens, or spring scenes.

2. Pass out a ball of clay about the size of a grapefruit and encourage participants to make a sculpture based on spring images they have seen or experiences they remember. This could be as simple as a nest with a bird and eggs or as complicated as a person in a garden.

3. Animal forms are fun to create and lend themselves beautifully to clay. Begin with a simple cylinder form for the body and add on head and legs.

4. An alternative lesson could be making a collage of cut-out animal photos with the participants drawing buildings, fences, animals, a sun, and stick figures.

AFTER

1. Display the sculptures in a central location where each creation can be viewed easily. (The clay sculptures can be saved and fired in a kiln or they can be put back into a ball, moistened, and saved for future use. A plastic garbage bag will keep the clay moist and soft for a long period of time.)

2. Ask the group what came to their minds while being creative. (The discussion might be tape recorded and replayed at a later date.) Help the participants to point out good features of each other's artistic and verbal expressions.

3. Ask if any of them are currently involved in nurturing someone or some living thing, maybe even a favorite plant? Discuss ways in which they can continue to care for and nurture each other. Ask what feelings helping someone else generates.

ADAPTATION

Clay provides an opportunity for highly satisfying manipulative experiences. If any of the group members has had limited experience with clay, encourage rolling balls, logs, patting pancakes, pinching, squeezing, pulling the clay apart, and sticking it together. Demonstrate when needed, a little at a time, the necessary techniques, such as how to score, press pieces together, and meld the newly attached pieces together for a permanent bond. Encourage familiarity with clay. Go to your local library and check out books on working with clay.

Creating a Garden Mural (Part 1)

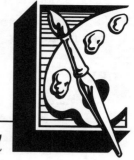

April

MATERIALS

- Long piece of white or brown butcher paper
- Pencils
- Oil pastels (or crayons)
- Block tempera paints
- Large brushes
- A variety of soil samples

BEFORE

Before gardening it is important to do warm up exercises to prevent muscle strain. Lead the participants in the following set of warm-up exercises:

1. Invite the group to stretch to welcome the sun. Direct them to reach as high as they can to touch the sun's rays.
2. Instruct the group to pick up imaginary shovels and press them into the soil, carefully bringing them back over their shoulders to throw off the dirt. Change hands and shovel another spadeful.
3. Direct the group to pretend to rake the soil smooth, reaching out as far as possible. With the toe, dig a furrow in the dirt to plant the seeds in. Change

feet and use the other toe. Suggest that participants sprinkle seeds into the furrows and stamp the dirt down with their feet.

4. Return to the first exercise in which the group stands up straight and reaches for the sun. Announce that the spring garden is ready for rain and growth.

Ask the group to discuss gardens they have grown in the past or are currently growing. What sorts of things did or do they plant?

DURING

1. Encourage participants to plan how they want to compose a garden mural. They may wish to use sketch paper at this stage.

2. Divide the group into people who want to work on the background and those who would like to create flowers, fruits, and vegetables for use in the mural later. (See note in the box at the end of this activity.) Individual tasks that can be designated include sketching the horizon line on the mural paper to delineate the sky from the soil, sketching the sun and cloud shapes, drawing leaves and vines above ground, adding color to shapes with oil pastels, and mixing appropriate paint colors for the sky and the ground.

3. After the mural is sketched, apply oil pastels for color and go over the soil and sky with block tempera paint. The pastels will resist the tempera and the paint will cover only background areas.

AFTER

Allow the mural to dry and talk about what you may want to add to the garden during the next lesson. Have the group make a list of favorite flowers and vegetables and ask anyone who can to bring in an example for the following week's class. Ask participants, "Is there a garden near you that you can enjoy?" "Is there a window box somewhere that you may be able to plant some things in?" An excellent follow-up activity to this lesson would be a field trip to a local nursery or greenhouse where participants can have direct contact with many types of plants.

ADAPTATION

This lesson focuses only on creating the background, but participants who are not able to work standing up can begin making separate fruits, flowers, and vegetables to place on the mural during the second phase of this lesson.

Creating a Garden Mural (Part 2)

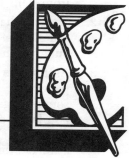

April

GOALS

- To reminisce about gardening activities
- To create a mural of a garden
- To focus on the senses of smell and sight
- To promote group interaction

MATERIALS

- Images of gardens from magazines such as *Southern Living,* books on gardening, and calendars
- Variety of vegetables and flowers
- Glue
- Scissors
- Various kinds of paper (colored construction paper, wallpaper, white drawing paper)
- Oil pastels, markers, and pencils

BEFORE

Look at the images of gardens. Present a variety of vegetables and flowers. (Participants may have things to share from their own or friends' gardens.) Urge participants to look closely at the colors and shapes. Ask what other sorts of things one might find in a garden (e.g., insects, scarecrows, tools, gardener). Ask what each person would like to create to "plant" in the garden mural. Group projects, in this case a mural, provide opportunities for those outside the group to become an integral part of the group by working together and getting to know the other people. Be sure to include newcomers in group projects.

DURING

1. Place vegetables and flowers around the room for visual stimulation. Have a variety of papers and drawing materials available for participants to choose from. This is a great opportunity for personal creativity—anything goes.

2. Suggest that two participants may like to work together to create a large squash plant. They can create large green leaves and yellow squash to cut out and glue onto the mural. They can also add insects to go on the leaves.

3. As flowers and vegetables are finished, lay them out on the background paper and arrange them thoughtfully before gluing them down. How will some things overlap others? If someone makes a scarecrow, where should it be placed on the mural? Think about every part of the composition. How are things above ground and below ground balanced? How are bright colors arranged throughout the entire composition?

AFTER

After participants have finished placing the flowers and vegetables on the mural, consider adding emphasis by outlining some of the shapes with a permanent black marker. How does everyone feel about the overall design? What else needs to be added? Encourage the group to decide together when they think the mural is complete. Display the garden mural on a wall in the facility. Perhaps participants/artists would like to have their photograph taken in front of the mural. They could give the photo to friends or family members.

Reminiscence and Improvisation

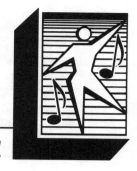

April

GOALS

- To reminisce about springs of the past
- To stimulate the imagination by translating memories of springtime experiences into movement
- To plan, create, and implement a group performance

MATERIALS

- Springtime pictures, such as pictures of spring flowers, baby animals, budding trees, blooming trees, spring rains, spring planting, spring fruits and vegetables, melting snow, Easter eggs, and so forth
- Cassette player and cassettes

BEFORE

Ask participants what they associate with spring. Pass the springtime pictures around. Ask what spring memories they would like to share. Let everyone share at least one spring memory.

DURING

1. Direct the participants to translate their memories into movement. Explain that they do not need to "act out" or pantomime the memory from beginning to end. They can select different parts of the memory to put into movement. The movements do not have to be literal; they can express in movement how the flowers smelled, what the rain sounded like, or what it felt like when the days started to warm up and the trees began to develop leaves. Smells do not really *dance;* yet, movement can convey the quality of fragrance. Encourage participants to concentrate on how the movement feels to them, not on how it looks to others. If participants seem to be self-

conscious, turn them so that they are facing in such a way that they cannot see others.

2. After 5 or 10 minutes, split the group in half and let each half watch the other.

3. Initiate a discussion about the activity. Did any movements stand out? If they wish, people may describe how they made a memory into movement.

4. Have the group select four to six movements from what they saw to re-create as a group. Encourage participants to choose movements that others performed or to volunteer their own.

5. Ask the participants whose movements were selected to teach their movements to the group. Give everyone enough time to master these movements. Set counts so that everyone takes the same amount of time to perform each movement. Put on some music that can be used to suit the counts you have set.

6. Divide the group in half and have each half stand on opposite sides of the room facing each other. Let the first group perform the first movement while the other group is still. Then let the second group perform the first movement while the first group is still. Then let both groups perform the first movement together. Repeat with the second, third, and fourth movements. Then let the groups perform the movements in sequence (the first group performing movements 1 and 3, and the second performing movements 2 and 4), and finish with the groups performing the four movements in order all together.

AFTER

1. Ask everyone to sit in a circle and share experiences. How did the movements feel? Did people feel that they could successfully translate a memory into movement? Did they feel that any of their movements captured a sensation or feeling especially well? Did moving in this way bring more memories to the surface? Share the memories with the group.

2. Memories added to an awareness of the arrival of spring create a strong groundwork for poetry. Ask the group to write a poem (and work on it throughout the week) that incorporates significant memories and dance movements shared during this activity with new experiences of spring that they have throughout the week.

ADAPTATION

Amazing poetry can be written by persons who use language in a nonstandard manner. Word confusion, such as the replacement of "humidity" with "humility," is one of the many ways that the poetry of those who are considered illiterate can rival or surpass poetry written by the literate in expression, interest, style, and sheer beauty. Because poetry does not require normal syntax or rules of grammar, it is much more accessible than prose or other forms of writing. For those who cannot write, a scribe can be assigned.

Designs into Movement

April

GOALS

- To stimulate an eye for design
- To heighten memory
- To use visual designs as inspirations for movement
- To translate everyday activities into movement

MATERIALS

- Paper
- Pencils
- Writing surfaces

BEFORE

1. Pass out paper and pencils.
2. Have participants sit down with a surface on which they can draw.
3. Ask participants to make a design of the path that they took to get to the room where they are now. The design should not be a map, but a line that represents their pathway. This pathway can begin in their rooms or at the front door of the facility.
4. When participants are finished (do not let this take too long), have them come together and share their designs.

DURING

1. Put all the maps together. Mix them up and let everyone pick one. Make sure no participants receive their own design.
2. Divide the participants into four groups of the same size. Direct each group to stand in one of the four corners of the room.

3. Ask one person to come from his or her corner and walk the path of the chosen design. Go around the room until everyone has walked.

4. Ask two people, from any two corners, to walk their patterns at the same time. Continue until all have walked.

5. Let the participants walk their paths whenever they like.

6. Divide the group in half and let each half watch the other as walkers come in on their own time. Let people come in more than once, making whatever variations they like on their design (e.g., designs can be smaller or bigger, turned inside out, curves can be made sharp, parts can be emphasized or minimized).

7. Return all of the designs to a pile, mix them up, and let the participants choose again. No one should have his or her own design or the design they picked before.

8. Direct the participants to explore movements that go with their new design. They may continue to walk the patterns on the floor, but direct them to move in more ways than just walking. Or, let them make the design in other ways, not in a pathway, but perhaps in other movements or shapes. Encourage them to make up as many variations as they can. Give them about 5 or 10 minutes to explore this.

9. Let groups of three people show the movements they have made to express their designs. When the participants have performed their movements three times, let each person show the design from which he or she worked to the group. Perhaps discuss people's choices after each group's performance, rather than waiting until everyone has performed.

10. Select one person's movement phrase from the performances. It should be a relatively simple and clear phrase.

11. Have this person teach the phrase to the group. When everyone has learned the movement, direct everyone to reverse it. Tell them they are to perform the phrase as if they are in a film that is being run through the projector backward. Let participants have the time that they need to figure this out (it is not easy!) and then let different groups of three share their solutions with the group. If people are baffled, demonstrate how to reverse a single, simple movement.

AFTER

1. Ask one participant to find an object or design in the room. The design may be handled or indicated by pointing.

2. Ask this person to create movements that relate to that design and ask the group to join in these movements. Allow a few participants to initiate this activity, then begin to end the session and ask these participants to tell how it felt to design a dance. How did the object or pattern that they picked help?

3. Discuss with the group what designs or instructions they follow on a daily basis. Suggest that the participants make up a dance at home or in their rooms that incorporates a favorite activity. During the next session, encourage each participant to perform his or her dance and let the group guess the nature of the activity.

Colors

April

GOALS

- To create movement from the image of colors
- To associate emotions with colors
- To participate in dyeing Easter eggs

MATERIALS

- Hard-boiled eggs
- Egg dyes
- Brushes
- Wax
- Easter decals
- Paper towels
- Bowls for the colors

BEFORE

1. Introduce color as a springtime motif. In spring, color re-emerges in the world. The dull grays and browns of winter give way to the colors of spring. Ask people of other ways that their senses (sight, smell, touch, etc.) "wake up" in the spring. What colors do people notice in the spring? (Answers might include: green grass, yellow forsythia and daffodils, purple violets and wisteria, red robin breasts, white and pink dogwood.) Spring is also the time to dye Easter eggs.

2. Distribute hard-boiled eggs among participants and let them choose a color to dye their egg. If you do not have enough time both to dye eggs and to do the movement activity, the egg dyeing could be done the day before and

participants could admire the colored eggs as a part of this discussion of springtime color.

3. Discuss how colors can show different moods. Let each participant have a chance to talk about the different meanings behind different colors (e.g., red symbolizes hot, and blue symbolizes calm). Begin a group discussion by asking questions concerning the mood that the color reminds them of and the feelings they associate with certain colors.

DURING

1. When participants have finished dyeing their eggs, and while the eggs are drying, ask participants to stand, if possible, so that they are facing any direction they like. They may hold onto the back of a chair for balance if needed. Remind the group that the purpose of this exercise is to experience what the movement feels like and not to perform movement they think others will want to watch. Encourage everyone to focus on how the movement feels.

2. Direct everyone to focus on the color red. Have them begin to move in a way that embodies red to them. If they like, people can throw out words that they connect with red as they move. Give people a few minutes to explore this color and then direct them to focus on the color blue. Continue through the spectrum in the same way: yellow, green, orange, purple, brown. Black and white may be included as well.

3. Have the group split in half and let each half watch the other.

AFTER

1. Begin a discussion of the number and nature of color choices in the immediate surroundings of the facility. Extend this discussion into the color choices they make in their daily lives (choice of clothes, choice of foods, choice of room colors). How do they account for the change of seasons in their decisions?

2. Invite the group to pay special attention to colors and their color choices during the coming week. Suggest that each group member take note of the most significant color choice that he or she makes throughout the upcoming week and share that choice and its significance with the group during the next activity together.

ADAPTATION

Persons with dementia may not respond well to inquiry concerning color associations. Chromatic identification and quantification, however, can provide challenge and enjoyment. Ask persons with dementia to point to all things that are red that they can see. Switch to blue. Challenge them to determine the number of orange objects in the room. Can they find the most rare or singular color?

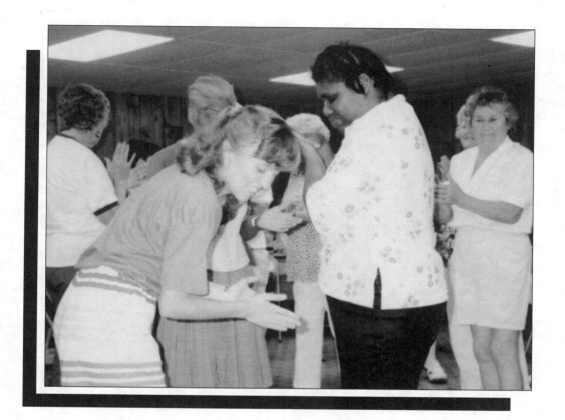

May

Themes:

Spring
Days of celebration
Friendship
Providing support
Sharing experiences

Springtime

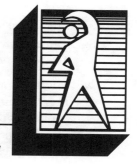

May

> **GOALS**
> - To promote cardiorespiratory endurance
> - To increase range of motion
> - To learn relaxation techniques

BEFORE

Talk with the group about signs of springtime. Have certain flowers bloomed? Do the trees show signs of new leaves?

Warm-up

State that everything seems to come alive when May arrives.

1. Walk briskly in a circle, or in place, carefully swinging the arms back and forth for approximately 2 minutes.
2. Alternate arm stretches overhead; hold each stretch for 6 seconds.
3. Facing into the circle, step to the side with the right foot, sliding the left foot toward the right. Continue moving right for several steps, then move left for several steps.

Breathe

Suggest that participants breathe as if smelling the flowers that are in bloom.

1. With hands on rib cage, inhale deeply and feel the chest expand (hands will move outward).
2. Exhale and feel the hands come closer together.
3. Repeat inhalation and exhalation 3–4 times.

Stretch

Neck: Invite those involved to visualize flowers with every turn of the neck.

1. Lower the chin toward the chest, feeling the pull along the back of the neck.
2. Lift the head up and look straight ahead.
3. Repeat lowering and raising the head 8 times, holding each position for 15–20 seconds.

Shoulders/Arms

1. Breathe in and lift the shoulders up toward the ears. Exhale and let the shoulders drop down. Repeat 8 times.
2. Slowly push the shoulders forward, up, back, and down. Reverse directions. Repeat 8 times.
3. Slowly lift the arms forward and upward; then drop arms. Repeat 8 times, lifting arms somewhat higher each time.
4. Alternately reach upward with right and left arms. Repeat 8 times.

Hands/Wrists

1. Place hands out in front and flex the wrists (raise fingers upward) then push down. Repeat 6–8 times.
2. Alternately open and close the hand. As hands are opened, stretch the fingers. Repeat 6–8 times.

Side/Waist: Ask the participants to feel themselves bend and stretch and feel more alive.

1. Standing with feet approximately 1 foot apart, raise the right arm over the head and bend the body slightly to the left. Return to an upright position and lower the arm. Repeat the exercise with the left arm. Continue alternating right and left arms 8 times.
2. Keeping the head in line with the upper body, bend forward as if bending over to pick a flower, then return to an upright position. Repeat 6–8 times.

Legs/Feet: Suggest that May makes one remember being allowed to go barefoot as a child after the cold winter months. Remind participants of how good it felt to run through the grass and feel the clover beneath their feet.

1. Holding on to the back of a chair, lift the right foot off the floor and bring the right knee toward the chest. Repeat with the left leg. Alternate the right and left legs 8 times.
2. With hands on the back of a chair, alternate lifting right and left legs out to the side. Repeat 8 times.
3. With shoes off and hands on the back of a chair, shift weight to heels and curl toes under, then evenly distribute weight on feet. Repeat 6–8 times.

DURING

Take the group for a 15-minute walk outdoors. Make sure that participants monitor their pulse rates.

AFTER

Refer to the discussion on progressive muscle relaxation in the Fitness section of Chapter 3. Invite participants to sit down and relax in the warmth of the sun.

1. Progressively tighten and relax each of the muscle groups in the body. The tension and relaxation will be done alternately, with 10–20 seconds spent on each phase. Concentrate on the following areas:

   a. Facial muscles

   b. Shoulders

   c. Arms and hands

   d. Legs and feet

2. After participants have fully relaxed, asked them to think of other thoughts that the month of May brings to mind.

SAFETY PRECAUTIONS

1. Encourage the use of the backs of chairs for support when lifting one foot off of the floor.

2. Alert participants to the possibility of uneven terrain during the walk.

May Day

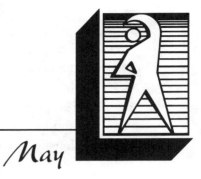

May

GOALS

- To increase flexibility through stretching exercises
- To improve aerobic capacity
- To develop muscular strength through the use of light weights

MATERIALS

- Beanbags, canned goods, and other light weights
- Cassette player and lively May Day–type music, such as "Waltz of the Flowers" or "Tip Toe Through the Tulips"

BEFORE

Have participants think back to previous May Days and how they celebrated them. Some participants may remember attending May Day festivals with carousels, relays, singing and dancing, and the winding of a Maypole. Suggest that they imagine attending such a celebration.

Warm-up

1. In a standing position, shake the hands loosely and then add the elbows and shoulders.
2. Holding on to the back of a chair for balance, shake out one foot and ankle gradually adding the leg. Repeat with the opposite leg.
3. Shake out the entire body and feel the warmth and tingling sensation.
4. Walk in place while trying to keep the body tall. Continue for 6 seconds.

Stretch

Neck: Encourage participants to visualize the sights of a festival with each turn of the head.

1. Turn the head to the right and then to the left. Hold each position 5–10 seconds.

2. Drop the right ear toward the right shoulder, then drop the left ear toward the left shoulder. Repeat holding each position 5–10 seconds.

Shoulders/Chest

1. With arms extended out to the side at shoulder height, palms facing forward, bring arms forward until hands touch in front of body and then return to starting position. Repeat 8 times.

2. With arms bent, hands in front of shoulders with palms facing forward, push arms out straight (parallel to floor) and return to starting position. Repeat 8 times.

Arms/Hands: Suggest that participants imagine dropping pennies into a bottle and tossing a ring around a dowel.

1. With arms extended in front of the body at shoulder height, make a fist with each hand. Open and close the fists alternately. Repeat 8 times.

2. With right arm bent and elbow pointed toward the ceiling, extend right hand toward ceiling until arm is fully extended. Repeat with the left arm. Continue alternating right and left arms 8 times. (This exercise should be done holding beanbags [or a light weight of some sort] in each hand. Each participant should have access to two beanbags.)

Side/Waist: Use beanbags or light weights with this exercise.

Standing next to a chair with feet shoulder-width apart and knees slightly bent, slowly lean over to the right. Return upright. Repeat 6–8 times. Repeat to the left side 6–8 times. Hold each stretch 10–15 seconds.

Hips/Legs/Feet

1. Position body next to a chair (using the chair for support) and swing the right leg forward, back, and forward again. On every third swing, hold the position for 10–15 seconds. Repeat with the left leg. Repeat 8 times with each leg.

2. Standing behind the chair, lift the right knee up and kick the right leg straight backward. Repeat with the left leg. Repeat 8 times with each leg. Hold leg in back for 10–15 seconds.

3. Standing behind the chair with weight on the left foot, turn the right ankle in a circular motion. Circle 4 times in each direction. Repeat with the left foot.

DURING

Ask the group to remember the relays at May Day events. Announce that they now have the opportunity to try one.

1. Divide the group into four lines. Explain that the object of winning is not to see who gets to the designated spot and back the fastest, but to walk briskly there and back.

2. Mark a designated spot in the room.

3. Ask all participants to walk briskly to the designated spot and back.

4. Repeat the relay several times.

Announce that it is time for winding the Maypole and for May Day dancing.

1. Ask the group to form two circles. The inner circle faces right and the outer circle faces left.

2. Begin the music and tell the two circles to march counter-clockwise for 10 steps, turn, and march for 10 steps.

3. Direct the group to move into one big circle and walk toward the center 8 steps, then back out 8 steps.

4. Facing the center of the circle, clap hands 4 times, then step right, step together, step left, and step together again.

5. Make a big circle with the right arm followed by a big circle with the left arm.

6. Walk toward the center of the circle for 8 steps and then back 8 steps.

7. Swing both arms up and down again.

AFTER

Suggest that May Day celebrations are nice, but rather tiring. Invite the group to cool down.

1. Swing both arms to the left and then to the right. Repeat 3–4 times.

2. Walk in place, gradually walking slower and slower.

3. Breath in and out slowly.

SAFETY PRECAUTIONS

1. Instruct participants to use the backs of chairs for support during hip and leg exercises.

2. Ensure that beanbags are in good condition to prevent stuffing from falling into an eye or causing unsure footing.

Friendship

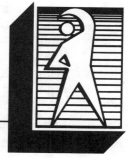

May

GOALS
• To focus on exercises that will improve balance
• To enhance joint mobility

MATERIALS

• Masking tape

BEFORE

Ask participants to think of friendship and the many things one shares with a friend. Before the lesson begins, place two parallel strips of masking tape 2 feet apart on all four sides of the room.

Warm-up

Suggest that everything we do is more enjoyable if done with a friend. A friend warms our heart and gives us a warm feeling all over. Ask participants to find a partner.

1. Tell the pairs to walk on the taped lines in a square around the room, inhaling and exhaling deeply as they walk. Repeat the walk 2–3 times depending on the size of the room.

2. Standing in place, swing arms upward and overhead and then down. As arms swing downward, bend the knees slightly. As arms swing upward, straighten the knees.

3. Wrap your arms around yourself and give yourself a big hug.

Stretch

Neck

1. Lower the head toward the chest and then raise the head. Hold each position 10–15 seconds.

2. Lower the right ear toward the right shoulder. Repeat with the left ear toward the left shoulder. Hold each position 10–15 seconds.

Shoulders/Arms

1. Extend arms at sides with palms facing backward. Keeping arms straight, raise the right arm in front of you as far above the head as possible and return to starting position. Repeat with the left arm. Repeat with each arm 8 times.
2. With the right arm bent and elbow pointed toward the ceiling, extend the right hand toward the ceiling until the arm is fully extended. Return to starting position and repeat with the left arm.
3. Extend arms down to sides with palms facing forward. Bring palms to shoulders and return to starting position.

Hands/Wrists

1. With both hands in front of the body about chest high, touch thumbs to each of the fingers on the same hand.
2. With both hands in front of the body, spread fingers, then bring them close together. Repeat 8 times.

Hips/Legs

1. With body positioned next to a chair for balance and knees slightly bent, raise the outside leg backward, making sure it does not go higher than the hips. Return to starting position and repeat 6–8 times.
2. Standing behind the chair with hands on back of the chair, raise the right leg upward so knee is at hip level. Hold 6–10 seconds and return to starting position. Repeat with left leg. Perform exercise with each leg 6 times.
3. Standing behind a chair with knees slightly bent, raise up onto the balls of the feet and hold. Return to starting position. Repeat 8 times.

Feet/Ankles

1. While seated in a chair with both feet flat on the floor, lift the right foot slightly and alternate flexing and extending the ankle 8 times. Repeat with the left foot.
2. While seated in a chair with shoes off, put both feet out in front of the chair and attempt to spread toes apart and then relax the feet.

DURING

Inspire the group to take a walk by suggesting that nothing could be nicer than walking with a friend. Ask participants to take a 15-minute walk outside with a partner. Heart rates should be assessed periodically during the week to ensure that no one is exceeding 120 beats per minute. The perceived exertion chart in Chapter 3 of this manual may be used to give a subjective evaluation of exercise intensity.

AFTER

1. Slowly stretch arms alternately overhead.
2. Standing on both feet swing to the right and then to the left. Repeat 4 times.
3. Walk slowly in place, concentrating on deep, slow breathing.
4. Conclude by asking the group to think of the many ways friendship may be expressed.

SAFETY PRECAUTIONS

1. Direct participants to use the backs of chairs for support for hip and leg exercises.
2. Move any objects that may inhibit walking.

Flower Garden

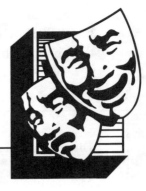

May

MATERIALS

- Pots for planting
- Soil
- Starter flowers
- Paper
- Pencils

BEFORE

1. Introduce the activity of planting flowers and experiencing the feel and smell of soil and flowers.

2. Assemble the group around a table. Begin a group discussion by asking each participant which flowers are among his or her favorites and what experiences he or she connects with those flowers.

3. Instruct the participants to pantomime the following actions, modeling the behavior as necessary. Tell the group to imagine that their favorite flower is in front of them. Tell the participants to pretend that they are actually smelling the flowers. Then tell them to pretend to feel its leaves and stems with their hands.

4. Ask participants to describe to the group what their ideal flower is like, to name its color, and to describe its shape and leaf shape. Ask them to tell what such a flower means to them and whether it is connected to a special person.

DURING

1. Distribute the planting materials and help the participants to plant their own flowers.

2. While the participants plant, ask them to be aware of the colors of the flowers and the feel of the soil. Suggest that they examine the entire plant, looking at the length and strength of the roots. Encourage them to smell the flower and stroke its petals. After they have experienced the flower thoroughly through touch, smell, and sight, encourage the participants to try sketching the flower.

AFTER

Begin a group discussion by asking each participant to discuss his or her plant, describing the flower's structure. Prompt each participant to describe what his or her flower looks like, how it smells, and what it feels like. Have each participant describe how it differs from his or her favorite flower. Urge each participant to tell the rest of the group where he or she might plant it or to whom he or she might give it as a present.

ADAPTATION

For participants with visual impairments, use plants that have definite tactile properties (e.g., the sharp edges of holly leaves, hairy stems of begonias, or a hollyhock's concave shapes). In fall, a locust tree's long curling pods are not only fun to feel, but also fun to shake. Mosaics can be made with seeds and dried beans, and floral arrangements can be made from dried plant life. Few natural objects give more tactile delight than horse chestnuts or buckeyes.

Mothers and Mothering

May

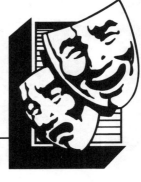

MATERIALS

- A bowl containing one kind of fruit (one piece for each participant)
- Gift-wrapped box
- Potted plant
- Chalkboard
- Chalk

BEFORE

1. Ask the group to talk about mothering. What do they feel are the qualities of motherhood? Make a list of these qualities on the chalkboard.

2. Ask each participant to name someone whom he or she thinks of as being like a mother to him or her. This person may be a friend, aunt, grandmother, stepmother, or sister. Write these people's names on the board.

3. Sometimes reminiscing can be emotionally difficult. Accept this as a part of sharing with the group. Give emotional support with statements such as "It must have hurt so much." Passing a box of tissues is a small way to show acceptance. Respect for the individual and empathy can help the person to cope.

DURING

1. Ask the female participants what they would like people to do for them on Mother's Day or Grandmother's Day. Ask the male participants what they would like to do to celebrate this occasion.

2. Suggest that the group act out their ideas about what they would like to have happen (or what has happened) to them on Grandmother's Day or Mother's Day. Instruct the group to take turns being the giver and the receiver. Is receiving also a way of showing love? Can anyone remember when someone was not willing to receive an act of caring?

3. Tell the group to think of a person who loved and cared about them and who helped them to grow up. Instruct them to think of all the persons in their life who gave love and helped nurture them to become the individuals they are today. These individuals can be teachers, caregivers, children, adults, and so forth. Encourage each participant to feel the warmth of all these "mothers" and to thank them for their love.

4. Divide the participants into groups of three or four. Have each person share with the group a mother figure in his or her life who made him or her feel loved and nurtured. Encourage each participant to repeat in a similar voice the things that person said to him or her. Tell each person to share a time with this person that was special. Ensure that each group has adequate time to share with the other groups.

AFTER

Ask participants if there is someone at the facility toward whom they act motherly. Ask the group to brainstorm ways of acting motherly. Encourage participants to act in motherly ways toward people at home or at the facility.

Conflict Resolution

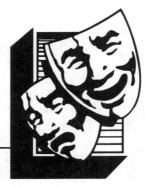

May

> ## GOALS
> - To recognize conflicts in the lives of the participants
> - To increase assertiveness skills
> - To act out conflict resolution

MATERIALS

- Chalkboard and chalk or large piece of paper and marker

BEFORE

1. Introduce the topic of examining conflict and finding resolutions. Help the group recall times when countries could not resolve their conflicts and the disputes eventually led to war. Describe to the group that conflicts between people can begin with uncomfortable situations, differences in values and beliefs, and differences in opinions.

2. Begin a group discussion by telling a story of how you were involved in a conflict with a family member or of how you resolved a conflict between members of your family. Then ask the participants to share with the group a memory of how they resolved a conflict or were involved in a conflict. Make sure all participants have a chance to state their conflicts.

3. Record on a large sheet of paper or a chalkboard the categories of the participants' responses. For example, list conflicts between brothers and sisters, parents and children, or cousins. List what the conflicts were about (e.g., privacy; sharing or misusing clothes, toys, or objects of meaning; being included or left out; freedom or limits).

4. Ask participants to offer strategies for resolving these conflicts, such as negotiating all aspects, being soft on the person but hard on the issues, or appealing to fairness.

DURING

1. Divide the group into pairs.

2. Allow each pair to select a conflict from the list. Tell each pair to prepare a skit about the conflict to present to the group. Each skit should contain a conflict and a resolution. Allow adequate time for each of the pairs to discuss and prepare their skits.

3. Gather the group in a semicircle to watch the presentations. Encourage the groups to clap for the performances.

4. Following each skit, inquire if others have had similar experiences and how they resolved their conflicts.

AFTER

Begin a discussion by asking the participants if they have any conflicts that are currently unresolved and that they would be willing to share with the group. To model such a discussion for the participants, the leader will probably need first to share a personal experience. Often, just acknowledging the conflict and sharing it with a group of other people motivates the person to think of a resolution to the issue.

Vases and Containers (Part 1)

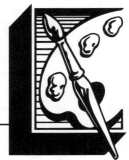

May

GOALS	

GOALS

- To create vases from clay
- To observe shape and form with containers
- To discuss uses of and experiences with containers

MATERIALS

- One pound of low-fire clay per person
- Burlap squares or newspaper
- Natural objects, such as twigs, leaves, or shells
- Toothpicks
- Small containers for water
- Bowls, vases, or other containers of various shapes and sizes

BEFORE

Bring in several kinds of bowls, vases, or other containers. Observe the different shapes and forms. Discuss with the group their round, cylindrical, square, tall, short, or fat forms. Discuss the ways containers are used. How does the shape of the container usually determine its use (or vice versa)? Who has a favorite bowl, cup, or vase? What does it look like?

The act of creating art can be therapeutic for persons who are lonely. The products present opportunities to give handsome gifts. Giving gifts of art to someone else can help with feelings of depression. At home or in one's room, clay vases filled with real or handmade tissue paper flowers can provide a cheerful addition.

DURING

1. Give everyone a ball of clay about the size of a grapefruit. Have a piece of newspaper or cloth for each person to work on so that the clay will not stick to the surface of the work area.

2. Demonstrate making a pinch pot. First, roll the clay into a smooth ball that fits fairly comfortably in the hand (about the size of a large orange). Using the thumb, press down into the center of the ball creating an opening. Rest the clay in the palm of the left hand and begin pinching the clay between the thumb and fingers of the right hand. Rotate the clay between each pinching motion gradually turning and working up the sides of the ball. Try not to leave too much clay at the bottom of the pot. The shape of the pot is controlled by the way it is pinched. It may be helpful to provide enough clay for an experimental pot before making the pot to be saved. This pot can be used for a flower arranging activity later in the month.

3. To add another design element to this project, textures and patterns can be created on the sides of the pot by drawing in lines and shapes with tooth-picks, or by pressing objects such as shells, string, or twigs (anything that has an interesting texture) into the clay. Advise the group to be careful to support the sides of the container as they do this.

AFTER

Display the finished pots so that everyone can view them. Discuss the variety of sizes and shapes. Did anyone have problems with the pinching process? How did it feel to work with clay? This activity is excellent exercise for the hands and especially good to combat arthritis. Encourage the group to think of other exercises they can do this week to strengthen their hands. Focus the discussion on uses for the pots.

Note

Allow pots to dry for at least 7–10 days before firing. If you do not have access to a kiln, ask a local potter for help or check with a nearby school to see if an art instructor would be willing to fire them.

Vases and Containers (Part 2)

May

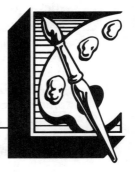

MATERIALS

- Pictures of painted or glazed containers or actual containers
- Books from the library on Chinese or Greek vases
- Block tempera paints and brushes or acrylic paints (Acrylic paints are excellent for applying color and designs to clay pots. They are water-based and adhere well to the surface of the container. If the art budget allows, purchase these instead of tempera at any art supply store.)
- Fired pinch pots from previous lesson
- Elmer's glue
- Containers for water

BEFORE

As a group, view the interesting patterns and color combinations in the different representations of pottery. Ask participants who brought in pictures or actual vessels to share their feelings or knowledge about the items.

DURING

1. Tell participants that they will be painting their fired pinch pots during this activity.

2. Provide each participant with a small container that has a 50/50 mixture of water and Elmer's glue, a paint brush, block tempera paints, and some clear water to clean the brushes.

3. Encourage participants to plan their design before applying paint. Do they want the inside of the pit to look the same or different from the outside? What kinds of patterns, such as stripes or polka dots, would they consider using? Do they need to paint a solid color first, let it dry, and then go back and add a pattern? Advise participants to dip the brush into the glue/water mixture and then rub it into the block tempera so that the paint will have glue added to it to increase its bonding potential.

AFTER

Allow the pinch pots to dry for several hours. They can be sprayed with polymer fixative if desired to add gloss and to protect the finish. Have the group share experiences about painting their pots. Ask why they chose the particular color and pattern they did. Where will they put their pot? Can they be displayed around the facility for all to enjoy? Do they have a friend or loved one to whom they might want to give the pot? Discuss how giving a handmade gift is a wonderful way to show love and friendship.

Creating Floral Arrangements

May

MATERIALS

- Images of floral bouquets (can be found at local libraries or in brochures available from FTD florists)
- Small scissors or clippers
- Clay vases from the Vases and Containers art activity (see pp. 180–183)
- Extra vases available for older adults who did not participate in the Vases and Containers activity
- Greenery
- A variety of flowers
- Florist wire
- Floral foam (green block of Styrofoam that holds the stems of flowers inside the vase)

Note

Local florist shops or funeral homes may donate many of the materials needed for flower arranging. In addition, some participants may have access to flowers and greenery that they can bring to the facility.

BEFORE

1. Stimulate a discussion of flowers and their meaning in the lives of the participants. Discuss why people enjoy growing flowers, what occasions often

involve giving flowers, and when participants may have given or received flowers.

2. Ask the group to look carefully at the flowers brought in for today's lesson. Encourage participants to notice colors, shapes, and textures. Ask the participants how the flowers smell. What memories do the smells trigger for the participants?

3. Display images of floral bouquets. Explain that flower arranging requires an artistic eye and lots of decision making. The Japanese are noted for their ability to create beautiful floral "compositions" and many people in this country belong to garden clubs that promote the art of flower arranging. Introduce the concept of creating a sculpture with flowers as participants prepare to make their own arrangements.

DURING

1. Hand out containers, foam, scissors, wire, and greenery.

2. Have participants fit foam firmly inside the vases.

3. Tell participants to attach the florist wire to the stems of the flowers and greenery and to begin placing the flowers in the foam. The first step in flower arranging and a secret to success is to cover the piece of foam as completely as possible with the greenery. Cutting the flowers to the proper size is also an important step. This gives participants the opportunity to exercise hand-eye coordination and to visualize the final composition as they plan their arrangement.

4. As they add flowers, encourage participants to turn their containers frequently to ensure that all sides look attractive. Tell them to think about the overall composition and consider: Which areas are too thin? Which flowers are so tall that they stick out? Are colors distributed in a pleasing way?

AFTER

After the memories have been rekindled and the arrangements have been made, discuss how these particular floral "sculptures" can be used. Perhaps the participants will want to give them to a friend or use them as a decoration for their room. An interesting follow up to this lesson would be to suggest that the group draw or paint their arrangements, creating a flat, two-dimensional representation that would serve as a reminder of the activity long after the actual bouquet has been discarded.

Reactions to Smells

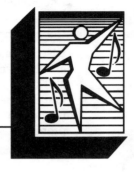

May

MATERIALS

For this activity, substances are needed that have a variety of smells: sweet, sour, bitter, memorable, pleasant, flowery, and so forth. The week before this activity, remind the group to bring these materials. Suggest that they pay close attention to smells throughout the week before selecting their material(s).

BEFORE

Choose about five or six participants to sit in front of the group. Pass one of the "smell items" down the line. Let each participant have a smell. Tell the group to watch how the participants react to the smell (focus on face and shoulders). Have everyone in the group "try on" the action that was a result of the smell. Make sure there is enough time for each smell.

DURING

Design a dance based on the group's "smells." Tell the group to express in movement the reaction to each material's smell. Allow the smells to become a sequence (e.g., chocolate, vinegar, cinnamon, mint, ammonia, chocolate, vinegar, cinnamon, mint, ammonia). Repeat this sequence at different speeds and levels of intensity. Let participants come up with variations. What happens when one smell meets another? What would the dance look like if all the smells were harmonious?

AFTER

Smells are known to bring about memories. Did any of the smells remind participants of the past or the present? Allow everyone plenty of time to share these memories and thoughts. Do other smells hold special significance to them? Have participants had an experience of smelling something they have not smelled for a long time and then remembering something or someone they had almost forgotten? If so, encourage sharing these experiences.

WARNING

Before implementing this activity, ask participants if they have any known allergies and, if so, avoid these substances.

Clapping and Moving to Rhythm

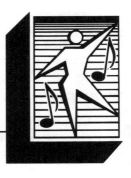

May

GOALS

- To make different rhythmic patterns by clapping and using movement
- To experience being a performer as well as an observer
- To develop cooperative and collaborative skills by sharing in a creative process

---

BEFORE

1. Invite the group to clap. Tell them to clap 8 steady counts, hold 8 counts, then clap 8 counts.

2. Ask one participant to hold (rest) for one or two numbers. (It is best not to hold 1 and 8.) Repeat the sequence with the holds inserted. Do this sequence several times.

3. As a group, walk the pattern and stop on the hold counts. While stopped, suggest that participants make interesting shapes. Do this several times. (The leader should clap so the participants can move. Try to encourage the participants to move all parts of the body.)

DURING

1. Divide the participants into two groups (A and B) and ask them to face each other. One group moves while the other claps (inserting the holds) and watches their peers.

2. Switch groups. Encourage the participants to work harder and experience "new" movement each time.

3. Switch the groups at least two times, then have the group, as a whole, do the sequence one last time.

AFTER

Ask both groups to come together and form a circle. Start a discussion about the activity. Discuss how the activity felt and how it felt to have peers observing. Share reflections about being observers and performers. Which role was liked by whom and why? Discuss the kinds of things that happen in life when we are interrupted and what we typically do when our routine gets interrupted. Ask what participants think they learned from this activity.

Allow time after the discussion for a cool-down with easy soothing music.

ADAPTATION

Persons who are challenged by movement may still be able to participate fully in this lesson. Members of the group in wheelchairs can move their wheelchairs around the room or they can move about in their chairs and be challenged to freeze at the appropriate times. Another option would be to involve the group or members of the group in more complicated clapping. Create a "Clap Orchestra," "World Beat Band," or "Hand Symphony." Participants can take on individual rhythms or provide a rhythm while others clap solo. Work with this group on syncopation (the rests and pauses in rhythm), dynamics (the loudness or softness of a clap), and orchestration (the way the overall song progresses).

What's Important?

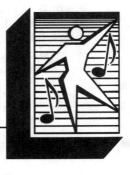

May

GOALS

- To provide an opportunity for creative expression of feelings
- To increase daily level of physical activity
- To focus on important and shared events

BEFORE

Have participants do the basic warm-up described in the Dance section in Chapter 3. Once completed, begin a discussion about the important factors in the lives of the group. What has happened in their lives that they feel is significant? What are some of the milestones or important events that have happened to or because of this group? What is important to the group?

DURING

1. Have participants pick four important factors in their lives and make movements to describe each factor.
2. Ask a few people to show their movements.
3. Suggest that everyone work together to make a group dance, using each other's ideas. Have each member of the group make a movement that describes something that is important to the group.
4. Select eight of the group moves and make a group dance. Repeat several times.

AFTER

Discuss the difference between personal importance and group importance. Ask questions such as:

Can something be important to you personally, but not to the group?

Can something be important to the group, but not to you personally?

What kinds of groups do you belong to?

What is important to those groups?

Are those things important to you personally?

Suggest that during the coming week, the participants spend some time thinking about things that are important to them, but not to a group to which they belong. Provide the opportunity in a later dance activity to share those feelings. Is there a group that addresses feelings that no other group in their lives addresses? If so, would they like to join that group? If not, would they like to form one?

ADAPTATION

If certain members of the group have a particular interest in sociology, literature, or history, or if they could be interested in one of these, suggest that a text be fashioned concerning the life histories of members of the group. Approaches may include interviewing a person and then transcribing the notes, or describing the effect that a specific event, such as the Depression or the assassination of President Kennedy, had on a person. Create a book of the final products and make copies for all to keep.

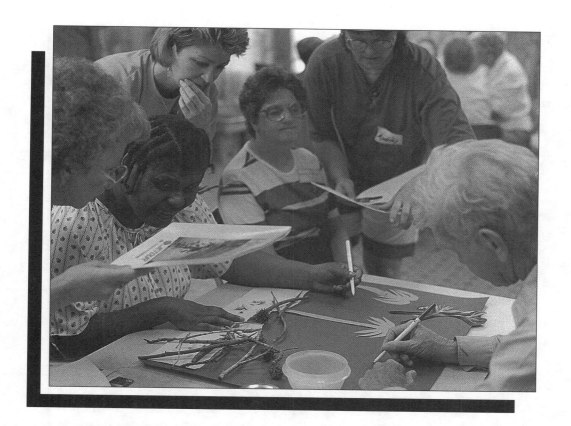

June

Themes:

Sports
Games
Fatherhood
Summer outings
Vacations
Relaxation

Summer and Vacations

June

MATERIALS

- Cassette player and cassettes of marching music

BEFORE

Announce that June has arrived and that it is time for vacations and summer fun. Ask the group what kinds of vacations they have taken and what kinds of activities they did on the vacations.

Instruct participants to use correct posture by placing their feet shoulder-width apart and standing tall, with hips rounded under, shoulders back, and stomach muscles contracted. To begin the activity, play marching music.

Warm-up

Suggest that the marching music will help get the group ready to enjoy the day.

1. Use the back of a chair for support, if necessary, and lift one heel off the floor, then the other heel. Lift only the heel, not the whole foot.
2. Continue to march in this manner and, if possible, lift one foot an inch or so off the floor. Repeat 8 times.
3. Continue to march in place while circling the shoulders. Repeat 8 times.
4. Stop marching and keep the knees slightly bent. If possible, release the chair and raise arms out to the sides and up overhead. Lower the arms. Repeat 4 times.

5. Lift arms up once more, this time reaching as far out and up as possible. Repeat 2 times.

Breathe

Suggest that when the group inhales, they smell the summer flowers in bloom.

1. Inhale slowly and exhale slowly two times.
2. Repeat step 1, raising arms to the sides when inhaling and lowering arms when exhaling.
3. Repeat step 2 while raising arms overhead then lowering them very slowly.

Stretch

Arms/Shoulders: Inform the group that when they stretch, they should release all their tension to really relax and enjoy their vacation.

1. Raising both arms up, reach one arm up, then the other. Repeat 6–8 times.
2. Roll shoulders front and back (6–8 times). Then exaggerate the movement by making the elbows lead the arms around. Repeat 6–8 times.
3. Stretch the right arm out in front of the body and grasp the right elbow with the left hand. Pull the arm across the body. Feel the stretch through the arm and shoulder. Repeat with the other arm. Repeat 6–8 times with each arm.

Neck

1. Drop arms by sides and stretch neck toward the left shoulder, then the right shoulder. Lower the chin toward the chest. Hold each stretch 10–15 seconds and repeat 8 times.
2. Turn head to look over one shoulder and then the other. Hold 10–15 seconds in each direction and repeat 6–8 times.

Wrists/Fingers

1. Roll the wrists in one direction and then the other. Repeat 6–8 times.
2. Wiggle the fingers one at a time, then touch each finger to the thumb. Repeat with each hand 6–8 times.

Legs/Ankles

Standing

1. With the support of a chair, slowly bend and straighten the legs, using the thigh muscles. Repeat 8 times.
2. Place one foot back behind the body in a calf stretch position. Make sure both feet remain straight ahead and flat on the floor. Switch legs.

Seated

1. Sit with both feet flat on the floor. Extend one leg out almost straight. Flex and point the foot. Switch legs. Repeat 8 times.
2. Repeat leg extensions, this time circling the foot in one direction and then the other direction.
3. Pull the right thigh up close to the chest to stretch the upper back of the leg. Repeat with the other leg.

4. With both feet flat on the floor, place the hands on the knees and slowly roll over and, if possible, place hands on feet. Slowly roll back up. Repeat once more.

DURING

Announce that it is time to get ready for vacation. Get the group excited about vacation by playing music such as "Those Lazy-Hazy-Crazy Days of Summer" by Nat King Cole.

1. Tell the group to take a walk on the beach. Swing the arms while walking along the shore. (Walk in place.) Look out at the ocean for sailboats. (Turn head side to side.) Throw an imaginary beach ball back and forth.

2. Tell the participants to take a hike in the mountains. Walk down the hills, bending the knees. Now walk up the hills, stretching on tiptoe. (Hold a chair for support.)

3. Tell the participants to practice throwing a baseball. Toss an imaginary ball back and forth. Throw with the left arm, then the right.

4. Ask the group to suggest other activities.

5. Have participants create their own movements to the music.

AFTER

Repeat warm-up stretches while gently swaying from side to side. Remember to go very slowly and gently. Stretch the neck, shoulders, arms, waist, legs, and ankles. Finish by reaching the arms high above the head.

Fishing

GOALS

- To increase balance
- To stretch and strengthen muscles especially, the thigh muscles (quadriceps) and the upper back and arm muscles

MATERIALS

- Cassette player and cassettes of relaxing music

BEFORE

To set the mood for fishing, play appropriate relaxing music. Announce that on a hot June day, nothing could be better than a relaxing afternoon by cool water. Suggest that with a fishing pole in hand, it is time to catch some supper.

Direct participants to use correct posture by placing their feet shoulder-width apart and standing tall, with hips rounded under, shoulders back, and stomach muscles contracted.

Warm-up

1. Sway from side to side using the back of a chair for support, if necessary.
2. Continue to sway from side to side, lifting each foot an inch or so off the floor. Repeat 8 times to each side.
3. Continuing to sway from side to side, lift one shoulder and then the other shoulder. Repeat 8 times.
4. If possible, release the chair and raise arms out to the sides and up overhead. Lower the arms. Repeat 4 times.
5. Stop swaying and lift the arms, reaching as far up as possible.

Breathe

Advise the group to inhale deeply and smell the summer flowers in bloom.

1. Inhale slowly and exhale slowly two times.
2. Repeat step 1 while raising arms to the sides when inhaling and lowering them when exhaling.
3. Repeat step 2 while raising arms overhead, then lowering them very slowly.

Stretch

Arms/Shoulders

1. Raising both arms up, reach one arm up, then the other. Repeat 4 times.
2. Roll shoulders front and back 4 times. Then exaggerate the movement by making the elbows lead the arms around. Repeat 4 times.
3. Stretch the right arm out in front of the body and grasp the right elbow with the left hand. Pull the arm across the body. Feel the stretch through the arm and shoulder. Repeat with the other arm. Repeat each arm 4 times.

Neck

1. Drop arms by sides and stretch neck toward the left shoulder, then the right shoulder. Lower the chin toward the chest. Hold each stretch 10 seconds and repeat 2 times.
2. Turn head to look over one shoulder and then the other. Hold 10 seconds in each direction and repeat 2 times.

Wrists/Fingers

1. Roll the wrists in one direction and then the other. Repeat 2 times.
2. Wiggle the fingers one at a time, then touch each finger to the thumb. Repeat with each hand 2 times.

Legs/Ankles

Standing

1. With the support of a chair, slowly bend and straighten the legs, using the thigh muscles. Repeat 8 times.
2. Move one foot back behind the body in a calf stretch position. Make sure both feet remain straight ahead and are flat on the floor. Switch legs.

Seated

1. Sit with both feet flat on the floor. Extend one leg out almost straight. Flex and point the foot. Switch legs. Repeat 8 times.
2. Repeat leg extensions, this time circling the foot in one direction and then the other direction.
3. Pull the thigh up close to the chest to stretch the back of the thigh. Repeat with the other leg.
4. With both feet flat on the floor, place the hands on the knees and slowly roll over, and, if possible, place hands on feet. Slowly roll back up. Repeat once more.

DURING

Announce that it is time to go fishing. Play music such as "Me and My Shadow."

1. Place fists one on top of the other, as if holding a fishing pole. Bring hands over the right shoulder and "cast" the fishing pole, extending out in front. Repeat to the left side. Repeat 8 times.
2. Practice reeling in a fish by bending over and straightening from the waist. Repeat 8 times.
3. Pretend to cast again, stepping out onto one foot. Return back to center. Repeat 8 times.
4. Cast out and reel in while repeating the step sequence above. Repeat 8 times.

Tell the group that they have caught plenty of fish and it is time to go home. Suggested music is "Marie."

1. Step side to side. Repeat 8 times.
2. Walk in place, swinging the arms front to back. Repeat arm swings 8 times.
3. Continue walking in place and extend the arms out one at a time, as though shaking someone's hand. Repeat 8 times.
4. Walk in place and reach the arms up one at a time. Repeat 8 times.
5. Walk in place and push the hands out in front. Repeat 8 times.
6. Return to stepping from side to side. Repeat 8 times.
7. Continue to step from side to side while swaying the arms. Repeat 16 times.
8. Finish by swaying side to side and rolling the shoulders. Repeat 8 times.

Instruct the group that more arm exercises are in order.

1. Practice casting the fishing line a few more times.
2. Lift elbows out to the side and bring hands in to shoulders and out again. Repeat 8 times.
3. To finish, shake the arms—really shake those arms.

AFTER

Begin a cool-down while playing music such as "Here You Come Again." Repeat warm-up stretches while gently swaying from side to side. Remember to go very slowly and gently. Stretch the neck, shoulders, arms, waist, legs, and ankles. Finish by reaching the arms high above the head. Give yourself a big hug, a pat on the back, and a big round of applause.

SAFETY PRECAUTION

Advise participants to use backs of chairs for support during standing leg exercises.

At the Beach

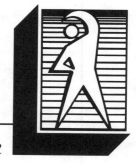

June

GOALS

- To increase strength, flexibility, and endurance and to continue to improve balance
- To develop cardiorespiratory endurance through aerobic activity

BEFORE

Ask the group to imagine that they have just arrived at the ocean. The tide is out and there is plenty of beach to enjoy. Urge them to think of the smell of the ocean, the feel of the sea breeze, and the sound of the surf. Suggested music is "Marie."

Remind the group to do exercises with good posture—feet shoulder-width apart, pelvis under, and stomach in.

Warm-up

1. Walk down the beach and back for a warm-up. (Walk back and forth across the room.)
2. Imagine standing at the edge of the water. Feel the cool water on the feet. Join hands and walk out a little farther. Stop and bend and straighten the knees.
3. Get ready to dive in!
4. Take both hands overhead and imagine pushing off and gliding through the water. Circle the arms forward as though swimming. Loosen the shoulders.
5. After backstroking back to shore (circle arms backward), shake the body to get some of the water off and then stretch.

Breathe

Raise arms out to the sides and take a deep breath. Slowly lower arms while exhaling. Repeat 4–6 times.

Stretch

Arms/Shoulders

1. Raise both arms up overhead and reach up first with the left arm, then the right arm. Repeat 8 times. Hold each stretch for 10–15 seconds.

2. Roll shoulders to the front, then to the back. Repeat 4 times in each direction.

3. Stretch the right arm out in front of the body and grasp the right elbow with the left hand. Pull the arm in close to the body. Hold 10–15 seconds. Repeat with the left arm.

Neck

1. Drop arms by sides and stretch ear toward one shoulder, then the other. Drop the chin toward the chest. Hold each stretch 10–15 seconds. Repeat 6–8 times.

2. Turn head to look over one shoulder, and then the other shoulder. Hold each position for 10–12 seconds.

Wrists/Fingers

1. Roll the wrists in one direction, then the other. Repeat 8 times.

2. Wiggle the fingers then touch each finger to the thumb. Repeat 4 times.

Legs/Ankles

Standing

1. With the support of a chair, slowly bend and straighten the knees. Repeat 8 times.

2. Place one foot back behind the body in a calf stretch position. Switch and repeat 4–6 times.

Seated

1. Sit with both feet flat on the floor. Lift the toes of one foot, hold 10–12 seconds, then lower the toes. Switch feet. Repeat 8 times.

2. Extend one leg and flex and point the foot. Repeat 8 times. Switch legs.

3. Extend one leg and circle the foot at the ankle. Repeat for 8 circles. Switch legs and repeat 8 times.

4. Grasp behind the knee and pull the thigh in close to the chest. Hold 10–12 seconds, then switch legs.

5. With both feet flat on the floor, place the hands on the knees and roll over slowly. If possible, roll over until hands are on the feet. Slowly roll back up. Repeat 4–6 times.

DURING

Now that the group is warmed up from the stretches, announce that they are ready to enjoy the day. Suggest that they move to music, such as "Sunshine," as if taking a stroll down the beach. (Try to keep the group moving for 10 minutes.)

1. Walk on heels for 8 steps, then on toes for 8 steps. Repeat 4 times. (If participants feel unsteady, they should stand behind a chair and march in place.)

2. Drag feet in the sand while walking 8 steps.

3. March in place 8 steps.

4. Walk back 8 steps.

5. Place feet shoulder-width apart and imagine swimming through the surf. Make big stroking motions with the arms. "Swim" forward 8 strokes and backward 8 strokes.

6. Step to the side and, if possible, sidestroke too! "Swim" 8 strokes to one side and 8 stokes to the other side.

7. Repeat steps 2, 3, and 4 until the end of the music.

AFTER

Inform the group that the swimming and walking on the beach was fun, but now it is time to cool down. Repeat the warm-up stretches after taking a few big breaths in and out. Stretch the neck, shoulders, arms, wrists, and legs. Finish with a big hug.

SAFETY PRECAUTIONS

1. Advise the group to use backs of chairs for support when doing standing leg exercises.

2. When doing the aerobic phase of the session, emphasize using support when the group is walking on their heels.

Movement

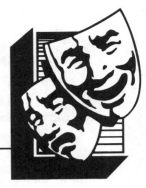

June

MATERIALS

- Chalkboard or large piece of paper
- Chalk or something else with which to write

BEFORE

1. Introduce today's lesson of celebrating the human spirit through sports and games. Ask participants to tell about a sport or game that they enjoy. These can be listed on a chalkboard or a large piece of paper. Include family games, such as badminton, croquet, and horseshoes. Also encourage participants to think of board games, such as bridge, gin rummy, and bingo.

2. Form the group of participants into a circle so everyone can watch each other do pantomimes.

3. Have each person pantomime a sport of game. Tell the others in the group to guess the activity. The leader's role is to lead the appreciative comments for each actor's clever way of showing the game.

DURING

1. Divide the participants into groups of four or five.

2. Allow each group to select one activity from the list and prepare a skit about the event. Urge them to think about what happens before the main

action and what happens afterward. The use of imaginary sporting equipment adds to the fun as the audience must visualize the equipment from the actor's cues.

3. To make the event exciting for the audience, encourage participants to develop dialogue for their skit. Suggest that participants concoct dramatic events, such as tennis balls flying over the fence and landing in poison ivy.

AFTER

Gather the groups in one circle. Have the group discuss whether people can succeed in an activity without "winning." Urge them to think about what really makes a person a winner in life. Encourage them to consider how they are each winners in life.

Some ways to extend the activity are as follows:

Direct the group to pick a favorite game that they would like to go see.

Inquire if there are games or evening activities in the community that participants might watch or join.

Ask if anyone would accompany a grandchild to a sporting event to cheer on the child.

Perhaps there is a nearby swimming pool where the older adults would enjoy watching the action of the children.

ADAPTATION

Persons who are physically challenged can enjoy participating in sports at the level at which they feel comfortable. To an onlooker this may seem to be far from the activity, but the imagination frees people from these limitations. Participation may be just holding sports gear on one's lap, waving a lightweight miniature bat, moving small boats in a shallow pan of water, or tearing out pictures of athletes from a sports magazine.

The Spirit of Fatherhood

June

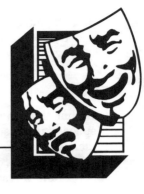

MATERIALS

- Chalkboard or large piece of paper
- Chalk, marking pens, or crayons

BEFORE

Introduce today's topic of remembering men who have loved and helped contribute to a person's growth and maturity. Ask all of the participants to tell of men who have been influential in their lives. Explain that biological fathers often cannot help raise their children because of extenuating circumstances; therefore, other people have the opportunity. These people might be a stepfather, an adopted father, a grandfather, an uncle, a scout leader, a teacher, a Sunday school teacher, or an older sibling. Record responses on a large sheet of paper or a chalkboard. Ensure that each participant has an occasion to share a memory.

DURING

1. Allow each person to choose a partner. Instruct participants to share with their partner a memory about this special person.

2. Ask each pair to create a pantomime about this special memory. One partner plays the role of the father figure while the other person plays the role

of the son, daughter, or young person enjoying the other person's attention. Allow adequate time for each pair to pantomime this memory.

3. Tell the pairs to change roles. Allow adequate time for all the pairs to pantomime their memories.

4. If some of the actors are willing to put on their skit for the entire group to appreciate, encourage them to do so.

AFTER

1. Ask the group to sit in a circle. Ask each of the participants to share a special memory about his or her father or father figure. Thank all participants for sharing meaningful memories with the group.

2. Query the group concerning how it felt to be the father figure trying to help another person. Help the group to determine what strategies the actors used in trying to be fatherly.

3. Urge participants to use what they thought about this activity throughout the week. Help them to think of someone in their extended family, neighborhood, or living facility who could benefit from "fathering." Suggest that the group brainstorm ways to provide the needed care or attention. Urge participants to give support to someone during the upcoming week and tell the group how it went at the next drama activity.

ADAPTATION

Some participants may harbor anger, rage, or bad feelings about their fathers or mothers. Substitute the words "people who have cared about you" instead of "father" in such cases. Should a participant want to give expression to such feelings, provide empathetic feedback. Acknowledge the value of expressing such thoughts and help the person to focus on positive steps for the future.

Picnics and Play

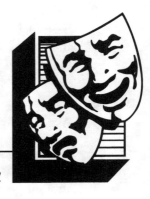

June

MATERIALS

- Chalkboard or large piece of paper
- Chalk, marking pens, or crayons
- Paper to cover tables

BEFORE

Introduce the topic of preparing for a summer picnic. Begin a group discussion by asking each of the participants questions such as:

- Have you ever been on a picnic?
- What did you bring to eat at the picnic?
- What other things are useful to bring along just in case something happens (e.g., bad weather, bugs)?
- What games have you seen played at picnics?
- What memorable things do you remember about picnics you have gone on in the past?

Make sure that each participant has a chance to respond to the questions. Record the responses on a large sheet of paper or a chalkboard.

DURING

1. Divide the participants into groups of four or five at tables.
2. Cover each table with a large sheet of paper for drawing.

3. Inform the groups that the table is their picnic spot. Explain that they will illustrate what their picnic spot looks like by making a drawing on the paper using marking pens or crayons. Have the groups consider including items such as trees, rocks, grass, or a lake in their pictures. Exciting, unexpected things such as rain clouds, bees, cows, and poison ivy might be included. Praise the way the participants are using colors and shapes to convey their ideas. Allow adequate time for the groups to develop their drawings.

4. Tell each group that an imaginary picnic basket is on their table. Have one person from the group "open" the basket and name the items in it while taking them out.

5. Allow each group to share what items have been taken out of the basket and to include them in the drawing. Ensure that each group has adequate time to draw these items.

6. Ask each group to name who is at their picnic and to describe what each person is doing. Inquire if anyone can recall games or pranks that are typically played at picnics. Encourage each group to describe the changing weather conditions.

AFTER

1. Ask all participants to sit together in a circle. Discuss how each group made its design for a picnic scene. Allow adequate time for each of the groups to present its picnic diagrams.

2. Begin a discussion by asking the participants what comes to their minds as a result of today's activity. Ask them to consider if picnics need to be held outdoors and far away or if they could be held indoors or outside the facility.

3. Help participants plan a picnic. Encourage them to think about what clothes they should wear and what activities they would like to do.

Architectural Designs: Field Trip

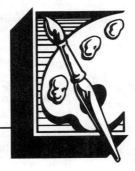

June

GOALS

- To enhance participant knowledge of architecture
- To promote community integration
- To increase observational skills

BEFORE

Plan an architectural tour of interesting buildings in the community with participants. The focus could be on downtown buildings, old restored homes, contemporary houses, or whatever outstanding architecture exists in the area. Perhaps a local architect or community historian would be willing to come to the facility to share his or her knowledge or to serve as a tour guide on the trip. Place photographs or posters of the community around the facility during the week to heighten anticipation.

DURING

The group leader or community volunteer can serve as a tour guide and point out buildings of interest. Encourage participants to look for certain architectural features and allow plenty of time for careful observation at each stop.

Activities to promote perception could be included. For example, plan a scavenger hunt with a list of interesting characteristics for participants to check off as they find them. Ask questions that encourage intense viewing, such as:

- How many triangles can you find on the facade of this building?
- How many arches can you find? Where are they?
- How many different materials can you name that were used to build this home?
- If this building could talk what would it say?

Perhaps some of the participants have memories associated with local buildings. Use this opportunity to reminisce about the past as well as to point out changes that have occurred in the community during the course of the participant's life there. The tour should be an appropriate length of time to accommodate the physical and mental stamina of the particular group. One person may be assigned to take photographs for everyone to discuss later.

AFTER

Consider stopping at a local cafe or restaurant for lunch or coffee to discuss the outing. This is a good time for the instructor to ask for feedback about the activity and what field trips the group might like to plan.

Architectural Designs: Drawing the Facility

June

MATERIALS

- Drawing paper
- Sketch boards (light-weight boards can be made from the backs of old wallpaper books or pieces of cardboard)
- Masking tape
- Pencils
- Erasers
- Folding chairs for use outdoors
- Cassette recorder and cassettes

BEFORE

Suggest that the group go outdoors, if weather permits, to take a close look at the facility and to create a drawing of what they see. If this is not feasible, use photographs of buildings that the group saw on the field trip in the June art activity "Architectural Designs: Field Trip" or other photographs of architecture as a motivation for the drawing lesson.

DURING

1. Encourage participants to describe what they see in terms of materials, general shape of the building, lines, patterns, and smaller shapes on the facade.

Look at the surrounding environment—the shrubs, flowers, and trees. How do they affect the look of the building?

2. Pass out small drawing boards with paper (if outdoors, tape paper to the board in two places to prevent wind from blowing it away), pencils, and erasers. Demonstrate how to draw the general outline of the building, gradually adding smaller details. Include any shrubs or trees that overlap the front of the building.

Because many participants feel uncertain about their ability to draw and to create art, *it is important for the instructor to move around the group during art activities giving encouragement and supporting all efforts.* Often, positive feedback can help artists overcome an initial reluctance, allowing them to stretch their perceptual skills and to achieve a sense of self-satisfaction. Focus should be on the process rather than the product.

AFTER

Exhibit drawings for everyone to enjoy. Utilize this opportunity for participants to reminisce and to share feelings about the facility and the friendships they have there. Tape record each person's memories, type them later, and display the typed transcript with the drawings.

Architectural Designs: Clay Tiles

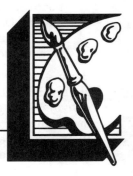

June

> ### GOALS
>
> - To create clay tiles
> - To increase awareness of architecture as an art form
> - To improve fine motor skills
> - To encourage use of the imagination

MATERIALS

- Images of unusual architecture
- Pencils
- Sketch paper
- One pound of low-fire clay per person
- Rolling pins (heavy cardboard tubes are good substitutes)
- ¼" lattice strips
- Burlap squares or newspaper pads
- Toothpicks
- Plastic knives
- Drinking straws
- Old toothbrushes
- Containers for water
- Glue and paints

BEFORE

1. Discuss the role of an architect as an artist who plans and designs build-ings.

2. Present visuals of interesting and unusual buildings from around the world—anything from the Taj Mahal to Buckingham Palace.

3. Discuss differences in architectural features and how the function of a building often determines its size and shape.

DURING

1. Ask participants to become architects and to design the facade of an imaginary building in clay. This could be the perfect long-term care facility, a dream house, or a fantastic skyscraper. Advise participants to do a quick sketch of their idea before they begin working with clay.

2. Pass out burlap squares, rolling pins, lattice strips, and grapefruit-size balls of clay to each participant. Working on burlap or newspaper pads prevents the clay from sticking to the surface of the work area.

3. Demonstrate rolling out a flat, even slab of clay. Begin by pressing the ball of clay down gently with the palm of the hand. Place the flattened ball between two lattice strips and begin rolling the clay gently with the rolling pin. Turn the clay when necessary to achieve the general size needed for the facade of the building. Keep the rolling pin on the lattice strips while working to prevent the clay slab from becoming too thin or uneven. Instruct participants to roll out their own slab.

4. Present plastic knives for use in cutting out the overall shape of the tile. Ask questions to stimulate the participants' creativity. What will the roof be like—angular or rounded? What is the shape of the building—geometrical or irregular? As participants trim away excess clay, they may want to save it to add shapes to the building later in the process.

5. After the general shape of the facade has been determined, the participants are ready to add lines, shapes, and textures. Extra clay can be rolled, patted, shaped, and attached by "roughing up" the clay with an old damp toothbrush at the place where it will be joined, then smoothing the pieces together with the fingers or with the tip of the plastic knife. Interesting details can be added by drawing right into the clay with a toothpick or pencil point. Encourage participants to incorporate interesting textures and patterns as they create their fantasy building. Shapes of trees, shrubs, and flowers can be overlapped in front of the building to add depth. The group leader should check that all pieces are well-attached so that nothing falls off during firing.

6. After the tiles are complete, have the group decide on their function. If they would like to hang them, they may use a drinking straw to make two nail holes. If this would present a design problem, they could glue a metal hanger onto the back after the tile is fired.

AFTER

1. Let tiles dry 1 week to 10 days before firing. Clay is very fragile, so the tiles should be stored in a safe place to avoid breakage during this time.

2. After the tiles are fired, let participants paint them with acrylics or with liquid tempera that has been mixed with Elmer's glue (three parts paint, one part glue) if they would like to add color.

3. Display the tiles around the facility for everyone to enjoy. These fantasy buildings provide the opportunity to talk about things to do to enhance the environment at the facility. For example: How would plants add color and beauty? What could be done to improve the interior space? How could the participants contribute to making the center an even more pleasurable environment?

Winds and Movement

June

GOALS

- To relax with breathing exercises
- To relive and share summer memories through words and movement
- To share personal experiences and favorite songs

MATERIALS

- Cassette player
- Nostalgic music—ask ahead of time that each participant bring in a song or select a song from the facility's audio collection that evokes a memory. The song need not be recorded; it could be sung or played on a musical instrument. Suggested music: "By the Sea," "The Summer Knows," "A Summer Place," "In the Good Old Summertime," "Think Summer," "Those Lazy-Hazy-Crazy Days of Summer."

BEFORE

Warm up the body to sunny, summertime music through breathing exercises. Raise the arms up overhead when inhaling, drop them down when exhaling.

DURING

1. Ask everyone to think back about an old summertime memory: a picnic, a wedding, a trip to the beach or another swimming spot, an evening on the porch, or just a special day.

2. Create a movement to go with the memory. The movement does not have to act out the story; it can describe other qualities of the memory: how hot it was, the fragrances of flowers, the shape of the porch, the motion or sensa-

tion of the water, the feeling of sweaty clothes, how funny a joke was, the sound of mosquitoes, or the taste of lemonade. A storytelling movement can be combined with a more abstract movement. Allow about 15 minutes for participants to complete their stories.

3. Let participants perform their stories twice. The first time, let the viewers share their responses and ideas about the movement. Then, ask the participants to perform the movement again, this time telling the memory during the movement. Compare the impact of the movement alone and the movement with verbal meaning.

AFTER

Invite each member of the group to sing or play the song that he or she brought. After each song, solicit feedback from the group. Ask the song's player to tell of the memories associated with the song.

Movement from Thoughts

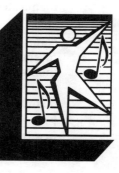

June

GOALS

- To enjoy a collaborative creative experience
- To share vacation experiences
- To explore cities through movement

MATERIALS

- Suggest the week before that participants bring in a vacation picture. These might include pictures of vacation spots (e.g., tropical islands, amusement parks, glamorous cities, one's own back yard); pictures of means of travel (e.g., planes, trains, boats, bikes, horses and buggies, campers); and pictures of activities one might enjoy on a vacation (e.g., sightseeing, touring museums, playing sports, eating out, visiting with family and friends, shopping, relaxing). Participants may bring pictures of themselves on vacation.
- Cassette player
- Music with a travel or vacation theme, such as "April in Paris," "San Francisco," or "Til We Meet Again"

BEFORE

Encourage everyone to describe a favorite vacation spot. Share vacation stories and pictures.

DURING

1. Ask participants to create movements to go with their vacation memories. Play some stimulating music, perhaps songs with traveling themes, and have participants enact vacation memories, such as putting on suntan lotion, grilling on an outdoor grill, or "swatting gnats."

2. Have the group split in half and let one half watch the other for a little while. Then switch the groups.

3. Bring the group together and talk about what everyone saw. Which movements stood out?

4. Have the group select four movements that they especially enjoyed. People can recall movements that they saw others do or participants can volunteer to share their own movements. Have the group rehearse the four movements together and then blend them into a phrase. The phrase might be structured like this: 8 counts of movement one, 8 counts of movement two, 8 counts of movement three, and 8 counts of movement four.

5. Play music and have everyone perform the phrase together. The leader may want to call out the counts at first. After everyone knows the phrase, have the group split into two groups. Let each group observe the other.

6. Alternatively, let participants choose their own four movements and combine them into a phrase made of 8 counts of each movement as above.

AFTER

Cool down to music. Imagine and discuss future plans for a vacation for the group or individuals, or dream up the perfect vacation. Prompt the participants to be creative and use their imagination in planning this vacation. Begin the group discussion with the focus on where they would like to go for vacation, how they will get there, where they will stay, what they will do when they arrive, and who will go with them.

If feasible, make this collaborative, creative experience a part of the facility. A display of vacation photos or exotic vacation menus, or a foreign film showing are some possibilities.

ADAPTATION

If the group includes persons who lose control of their temper, discuss heat and the month of June in relation to irritability. It is said that when the temperature is 93°F or higher, people are especially prone to anger. Modify the "During" activity so that the group creates movements that represent anger. Then move into the vacation or relaxation movements. Bring the two types of movements together in the dance. In the "After" activity, discuss ways of controlling anger: humor, physical activity, rest and relaxation, and hobbies or other activities that take one's mind off of the problem. Ask the group how vacations help people to curb their tempers. How can just thinking about a vacation help?

Baseball Movements

June

GOALS

GOALS

- To remember experiences playing or watching baseball
- To explore stretching, twisting, reaching, bending, and other movements
- To have the experience of transforming one movement into another movement
- To make dance out of life movements
- To enjoy exploring, performing, and watching movement

MATERIALS

- Sports pictures
- Gloves
- Balls
- Baseball caps
- Cassette player and upbeat music

(Both the leader and the participants may provide some of these items.)

BEFORE

Ask who has played baseball and who has been to a game. Ask if any of the participants is a baseball fan. Encourage the participants to share baseball stories.

DURING

1. Ask participants what kinds of movements are made in baseball. Let participants suggest and demonstrate movements and then have everyone do them together. Movements might include: swinging a bat, throwing a ball,

pitching, putting one's arms out and reaching to slide into a base, getting ready to steal a base, putting one's glove down to field a ball, putting one's arms up to signal catching a fly, or stretching out to catch a throw while keeping one foot on the base. Talk through these movements and give participants time to explore them.

2. Pick four movements and ask participants to perform them to music, doing 8 counts of each movement. Have the group split into two groups and watch each other.

3. Explore how the movements might be done with other body parts. Let participants explore this and then have them do 8 counts of each movement to music adding one or more body parts. Again divide the group into half.

4. See what happens when the movements are speeded up, slowed down, or turned into shapes. Again, let the dancers explore this to music and then perform 8 counts of each movement, using whatever combination of speeds they like. Have the participants split and trade watching and doing.

5. Ask the group to agree on what movements they liked the best. Everyone could learn these movements and do them together to music.

AFTER

Discuss how the movements changed. Begin the group discussion by asking participants if they felt like they were dancing when they altered the baseball movements. Suggest that the group take a field trip to watch a Little League game in the community. Inspire them with the thought of hot dogs, soft drinks, bright lights, and the cheering of the crowd.

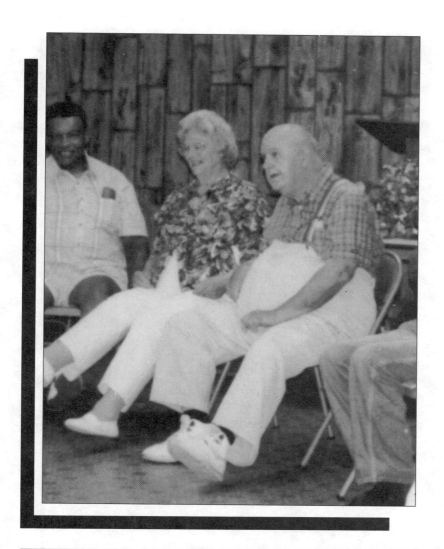

July

Themes:
Patriotism
Flags and fireworks
Altruism

Summer Olympic Games

July

MATERIALS

- Batons made of rolled paper with rubber bands holding them together
- Cassette player and cassettes

BEFORE

Ask participants to imagine that they are at the opening of the Summer Olympics. It is a beautiful, warm day. Suggest that they visualize all the activity as they warm up and prepare for the games. (Narrate this activity.) If possible, play the Olympic theme or music with a triumphant sound, such as "Chariots of Fire."

Warm-up

1. Ask each participant to choose a country to represent. Ask participants to move their feet up and down while either marching or sitting in place. This keeps the excitement alive while representing each country in the Olympics.

2. As the countries enter the arena, all participants will march around the area. Seated participants use their arms while "marching."

3. Face the inside of the circle and join hands.

Stretch

1. Step a little closer and relax the shoulders, releasing the hands.

2. Stretch the neck to one side, the other, and down in front. Repeat 4–6 times.

3. While maintaining good body position (knees relaxed, pelvis tucked), turn the head to see the neighbor to the right, then turn to see the neighbor to the left.

4. Raise arms in front and walk forward until all participants' hands are clasped in the middle. Seated participants should begin this handmade knot.

DURING

1. Relay races: Divide the participants into four groups and form a line either standing or seated. Practice passing a baton from one person to the next. Pass the baton up and down the lines.

2. Swim: Direct the group to make big arm circles, first to the front, then to the back, as though they were swimming in a meet.

AFTER

1. Cool down by coming together in the center of the circle and joining hands.

2. Sway from one side to the other, holding hands.

3. Step forward and backward, bringing arms front and back.

ADAPTATION

All warm-up and stretching exercises may be performed in a seated position by participants who are unable to stand. Persons in wheelchairs may swing arms instead of marching, and may roll their wheelchairs forward when walking is designated. Relay races may be done in a seated position.

A Parade

July

MATERIALS

- Cassette player and cassettes of patriotic music

BEFORE

Announce that the Fourth of July marks American independence. Encourage the participants to celebrate during the session. Tell participants that this activity is a marching parade. Suggested music is "I'm a Yankee Doodle Dandy." Direct participants to use correct posture:

1. Stand with feet shoulder-width apart.
2. Bend knees slightly and tuck pelvis under.
3. For those participants who are seated, press the lower back into the seat and contract the abdominal muscles.

Warm-up

1. Bringing the feet up and down, march in place (standing or seated).
2. Carefully swing the arms back and forth while marching in place.
3. Stand up tall and continue marching in place until the end of the music.

Stretches

Arms/Shoulders

1. Raise both arms overhead and reach up first left, then right. Repeat 8 times.

2. Roll shoulders to the front and to the back. Repeat 4 times in each direction.

3. Stretch the left arm out in front of the body and grasp it by the elbow with the right hand. Pull the arm in close to the body. Repeat with the right arm. Repeat 4–5 times with each arm.

Neck

1. Drop the arms and lower the head toward the left shoulder, then toward the right shoulder. Drop the chin toward the chest. Repeat each position 4 times.

2. Turn the head to look over one shoulder and then the other.

Wrists/Fingers

1. Rotate both wrists in one direction, then the other. Repeat 8 times in each direction.

2. Wiggle the fingers. Touch each finger to the thumb. Repeat 2 times with each hand.

Legs/Ankles

Standing

1. With the support of a chair, slowly bend and straighten the knees. Repeat 8 times.

2. Place the right foot back in the calf stretch position. Repeat with the left foot.

Seated

1. Sit with both feet flat on the floor. Lift the toes of one foot, then the other. Repeat 8 times.

2. Extend one leg and flex and point the foot 8 times. Switch legs.

3. Extend the right leg and circle the foot at the ankle 8 times. Repeat with the left leg.

4. Grasp behind the right knee and pull the thigh close to the chest. Repeat with the left leg.

5. With both feet flat on the floor, place the hands on the knees and roll forward slowly. If possible, roll forward until hands are on feet. Slowly roll back up. Repeat.

DURING

Announce that the parade will begin now. Suggest that everyone pretend to have some sort of instrument—a trombone, a drum, or cymbals. The idea is to step in a lively manner and enjoy this national celebration. Suggested music is marching music, such as "Stars and Stripes Forever" or "Washington Post March."

1. March in place for 16 counts. Repeat left, right, left, right, and so on.

2. March in place for 16 counts with knees high.

3. March forward 8 steps, in place 8 steps, backward 8 steps, and in place 8 steps. Repeat 4 times.

4. March forward 8 steps, in place 8 steps, turn right a quarter turn, and march in place 8 steps and repeat. Continue to make a square. Repeat step 3 until music stops.

5. Begin music (preferably another song) and repeat the march sequence in steps 1–4, adding arm movements by imitating instruments. If the idea of instruments does not work, have the "marchers" use their arms in some other fashion.

AFTER

Suggest that after so much marching, it would be a good idea to walk slowly around the room. Positively recap the experience of the parade. Remind the group to drink lots of water during these summer days.

1. Repeat each of the stretches at the beginning of the activity 2 times, taking a few deep breaths in and out.

2. Finish the cool-down by asking the participants to give themselves or each other a big hug.

Fireworks and a Fourth of July Celebration

July

GOALS

- To increase strength, flexibility, and cardiorespiratory endurance by participating in activities related to a summer celebration
- To have fun celebrating a national holiday

MATERIALS

- Cassette player and cassettes of patriotic music

BEFORE

State that the Fourth of July marks the independence of this nation, but it can also be a time to celebrate the independence of individuals. Introduce this activity as a walk in a park to watch a beautiful fireworks display. Suggested music is "The Star-Spangled Banner." Direct participants to use correct posture:

1. Stand with feet shoulder-width apart.
2. Bend knees slightly and keep pelvis tucked.
3. For those seated, press the lower back into the rear of the seat and contract the abdominal muscles.

Warm-up

Suggest that the group imagine that they are in a park on a summer evening. As the sun is setting, everyone is becoming excited about the upcoming fireworks display.

1. Move feet up and down while walking or sitting in place.
2. Carefully swing arms back and forth while marching in place.
3. Stand up tall and continue marching in place until the music stops.

Stretch

Arms/Shoulders

1. Raise both arms overhead and reach up higher with the left arm, then the right arm. Repeat 8 times.
2. Roll the shoulders to the front, then to the back. Repeat 4 times in each direction.
3. Stretch the left arm out in front of the body and grasp it by the elbow with the right hand. Pull the arm in close to the body. Repeat with the right arm.

Neck

1. Drop arms by sides and stretch head toward one shoulder, then the other. Then drop the chin toward the chest.
2. Turn head and look over one shoulder and then the other.

Wrists/Fingers

1. Roll the wrists in one direction, then the other. Repeat 8–10 times in each direction.
2. Wiggle the fingers. Touch each finger to the thumb. Repeat 2 times.

Legs/Ankles

Standing

1. With the support of a chair, slowly bend and straighten the knees. Repeat 8–10 times.
2. Place one foot in back in the calf stretch position. Switch feet.

Seated

1. Sit with both feet flat on the floor. Lift the toes of one foot, then the other. Repeat 8–10 times.
2. Extend one leg and flex and point the foot 8 times. Switch legs.
3. Extend one leg and circle the foot at the ankle 8 times. Switch legs.
4. Grasp behind one knee and pull the thigh in close to the chest. Switch legs.
5. With both feet flat on the floor, place the hands on the knees and roll forward slowly. If possible, roll forward until the hands are on the feet. Slowly roll back up. Repeat.

DURING

Tell the participants to prepare for the fireworks. The fireworks will be created when participants imitate explosions with their arms. Remember, this is a festive occasion. Try to keep moving for 10 minutes. Have the group form a circle. Suggested music for this activity is "106 Trombones" from "The Music Man."

1. Walk in place, lifting the heels off the floor for 16 counts. Say "left" and "right" aloud while lifting heels.
2. Walk in place, pushing heels down in front of the body for 16 counts.

3. Walk forward 8 steps, in place 8 steps, backward 8 steps, and in place 8 steps. Repeat 4 times.

4. Walk forward 8 steps while sweeping the arms overhead. At the center of the circle, stretch the fingers out to imitate fireworks exploding overhead. Walk backward and lower the arms to the sides. Repeat this sequence 4 times.

A second activity for arm movement is the "wave."

1. Maintain the circle and walk in place, swinging the arms from front to back. Repeat 16 times.

2. Place feet shoulder-width apart and sway the arms from side to side, rocking from one foot to the other. Repeat 16 times.

3. Begin with one person raising then lowering his or her arms and make a "wave" all the way around. Repeat 4 times.

4. Repeat the "wave" in the other direction.

5. Finish the dance by raising the arms overhead while walking into the center 8 steps; push the arms down while walking back 8 steps. Repeat until the end of the song.

AFTER

Announce that now it is time to cool down.

1. Repeat the stretches at the beginning of the activity after taking a few deep breaths in and out.

2. Finish with a big hug.

Patriotism and Individual Rights

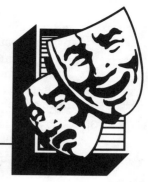

July

GOALS

- To stimulate cognitive functioning
- To increase nonverbal communication skills
- To encourage spontaneous expression of feelings

BEFORE

Begin the lesson by introducing the themes of the Fourth of July and patriotism. Describe what the Fourth of July and patriotism mean to you, the leader. Then, initiate a group discussion by asking participants to tell what the Fourth of July and patriotism mean to them. Make a list of what participants believe the government does for them. What rights does this country guarantee its citizens? Also, make a list of what an individual owes to his or her country. Discuss if there are times when an individual disagrees with something his or her country is doing. Discuss how the founders of this country often disagreed.

DURING

1. Divide the participants into groups of four or five. Members in each group will discuss events or activities that make them feel patriotic. Each group will select one member's event or activity to pantomime. Examples might include enacting a row of drummers or buglers in a parade; setting off fireworks; going to war, to boot camp, or to work in a factory involved in the war effort; raising a victory garden; or writing one's congressional representative about legislation that should be passed.

2. Allow adequate time for each of the groups to discuss and rehearse their pantomimes. Ask all of the participants to form a semicircle.

3. Have each group perform its skit while everyone watches.

AFTER

1. Help the participants think of names for each of the skits they saw.

2. To assist the group members to extend this activity into their lives, discuss good ways to spend the Fourth of July. Ask those participants who will watch a parade or see fireworks to discuss what they will see. Ask if anyone is planning to go on a picnic or watch fireworks on television. Brainstorm together about ways that such events could be more fun. Perhaps there are special foods that might be purchased, such as marshmallows or hot dogs.

3. Ask participants who cook or who recall cooking to share a favorite potato salad recipe or cole slaw recipe that can be used on picnics.

4. Inquire if there are any activities that participants did as children on the Fourth of July that might be shared with grandchildren and other children today.

5. Thank the participants for making this Fourth of July celebration special and meaningful.

Yankee Doodle Dandy

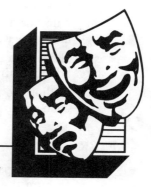

July

GOALS

- To encourage spontaneous expression
- To encourage recall of melodies and songs
- To increase the level of physical activity with the hands and arms

---

MATERIALS

- Cassette player
- Cassette of patriotic songs, including "Yankee Doodle Dandy"
- Photocopies of the lyrics to "Yankee Doodle Dandy"

BEFORE

Gather the group into a circle. Explain that the group will use four actions as part of the exercise. Tell the participants that when they hear the word "pat," they will pat their thighs with the palms of their hands. When they hear the word "clap," they will clap their hands together. When they hear the word "snap," they will snap their fingers. When they hear the word "shuffle," they will shuffle their feet on the floor. During this exercise play the song "Yankee Doodle Dandy." Have the group practice these four movements together as a way of loosening their muscles.

DURING

1. Begin with a simple pattern, such as pat-pat-clap-clap-snap-snap. Continue with this pattern until the words and actions are coordinated.
2. Pass out the words to the song "Yankee Doodle Dandy."

3. Begin the music and tell the group to begin singing "Yankee Doodle Dandy" while they shuffle. Ask if one or two participants might be interested in taking turns leading the group.

4. Another activity is to divide the participants into groups of three or four and ask each group to discuss the lyrics of "Yankee Doodle Dandy."

5. Have each group improvise a skit that follows the words of the song. Allow adequate time for the groups to discuss the song and develop their skit.

6. Gather the groups into a semicircle. Play the song at a soft volume while each group performs.

AFTER

1. Help the participants recall other favorite patriotic songs. Encourage them to hum the rhythms or sing any words that they can remember. "You're a Grand Old Flag," "America," "My Country 'Tis of Thee," and "The Star-Spangled Banner" are some that may be familiar.

2. Play a record or cassette of patriotic songs so that everyone can sing along.

3. Encourage participants to recall any special times when they heard such songs, or special times in their lives when their patriotism was put to the test. You might tell a story about a time when you heard such songs and were moved by the sentiment.

4. Someone may want to share an anecdote about going to war or having a loved one go to war.

A Picture Is Worth a Thousand Words

July

GOALS

- To increase social interaction skills
- To increase attention span
- To stimulate cognitive functioning
- To understand that limitations do not prevent participation

MATERIALS

- Paper
- Pencils or markers

BEFORE

Introduce this activity of turning words into pictures and then turning pictures back into words. Just as the game "Charades" requires communicating without words, this activity also involves communicating without words. For those who have played the game "Pictionary," this sort of activity, involving communicating through sketching, will be familiar.

DURING

1. Divide the participants into two groups. Tell each group to choose things or actions for the other team to draw.
2. Tell each group to write the name of each object or action on a card or small piece of paper.
3. Ask one person to pick one of the cards from the opposite group, show it to the group that wrote it, sketch it, and then pantomime it for his or her own

group. When drawing, do not use any words except "yes" and "no" to communicate to the group.

4. Tell the person's group to try to guess the word or action in as short an amount of time as possible.

5. Play should continue until each person in the group has a chance to draw and then pantomime for his or her group.

AFTER

Begin a group discussion by asking how difficult communication was without words. Inquire if anyone knows of someone who communicates by using alternative methods such as gestures and pictures. Encourage the participants to tell stories about how people they know have overcome challenging circumstances. Discuss how people use alternative ways for speaking, hearing, remembering, and mobility. Perhaps someone would be willing to tell about his or her own discouragement and then strength in overcoming a challenging condition. Discuss how an attitude of "can do" makes the difference. Thank the group for their participation.

Fireworks Mural

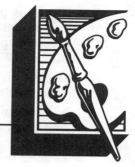

July

MATERIALS

- Images of fireworks displays from magazines or fireworks catalogs
- Long sheet of white bulletin board paper
- Oil pastels
- Watercolors or cake tempera
- Brushes
- Containers for water
- Glue
- Glitter
- Foil

BEFORE

1. Present visuals of fireworks and discuss past Fourth of July holidays. Ask the group how they have celebrated this occasion. What do they remember about seeing fireworks?

2. Ask members of the group to pretend to describe fireworks to someone who has never seen them.

3. Have the group make a list of words to describe fireworks. What colors do they come in? What shapes are they? Do the participants like the noisy kind or the beautiful kind?

4. Announce that the group will make a mural of a sky full of fireworks.

DURING

1. Spread out a long sheet of white paper on a table and have participants sit on all sides.

2. Direct the participants to use oil pastels to create colorful fireworks, thinking about the colors and shapes that have been described. Encourage a fairly heavy application of pastels. One color can be placed on top of another and blended.

3. Suggest that members of the group add foil cutouts of stars, comets, and glittering fireworks by gluing them to the mural.

4. After the mural is covered with shapes and colors, instruct participants to do a "wash" over the pastels and collage shapes for the sky. An application of black or dark blue block tempera paint over the entire mural will provide a strong contrast to the bright fireworks. Advise clients to keep the paint application light and diluted in order not to cover the pastels.

5. After the background is dry, have participants look thoughtfully at the mural. Consider how all parts of the composition are balanced. What area needs more shapes or brighter colors? Pastels or foil shapes can be added there. Another way to create the effect of fireworks is by drawing lines and shapes on the background with glue and then sprinkling glitter on top.

AFTER

1. Talk about the process of making the mural. What did the participants enjoy most about working as a group on this project? How did they help each other? At what other times are they involved as a group at the facility?

2. Ask the group to decide where to hang the Fourth of July mural for all to enjoy. This could become a backdrop for a drama activity or motivation for singing some patriotic songs, such as "You're a Grand Old Flag" or "My Country 'Tis of Thee."

Flags: Designing a Banner (Part 1)

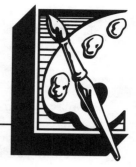

July

MATERIALS

- Flags or books with illustrations of flags
- White drawing paper
- Pencils
- Markers
- Rulers

BEFORE

1. Show participants a variety of flags and books with illustrations of flags. It would be interesting to have images of the American flag as it evolved from the original Betsy Ross version to its present form.
2. Discuss the meaning of shapes on flags.
3. Invite the group to look at the state flag. What shapes and symbols does it contain? What are their meanings?
4. Ask participants what it was like to fly a flag of their own, perhaps one that they displayed at their home. What kind of significance does the flag have for them?
5. Ask participants to share a memory with the group that involves a flag.

DURING

1. Pass out sheets of white drawing paper, pencils, rulers, and markers.

2. Ask participants to think about a design for a banner that would represent the facility. Is there something that is unique about the building that could be incorporated as a shape or symbol? Maybe there is a beautiful tree or plantings that participants have noticed. Each individual could create a personal symbol to become a part of the banner.

3. Instruct participants to plan what colors will be used and draw out individual designs.

AFTER

Display the banner designs and ask participants to share the meanings of their particular symbols as they relate to the facility. Have the group think about choosing one design or a combination of several designs for Part 2 of this lesson on painting a large banner for the facility. If individual symbols have been created, then all of them can be incorporated into the finished product.

ADAPTATION

Encourage participants with and without disabilities to work together on their designs. For example, if a person with mental retardation enjoys softball, he or she could work together with a person without disabilities who has the same interest. The work can be signed by both people.

Flags: Designing a Banner (Part 2)

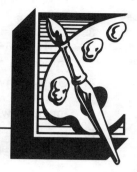

July

GOALS

- To paint a banner for the facility
- To gain awareness of symbolism in flags
- To understand elements of design in flags
- To foster group decision-making skills
- To create a composite design based on individual designs

MATERIALS

- Large piece of white bulletin board paper
- Pencils
- Block tempera paints
- Brushes
- Containers for water
- Glue
- Scissors
- Permanent markers and/or oil pastels

BEFORE

Review the July art lesson, "Flags: Designing a Banner (Part 1)." Have participants decide how they want to combine the designs they created during that lesson into a large banner for the facility. This is a good opportunity to allow the group to work together. Offer several alternatives—the group can vote on one design that they think best represents the facility, they can decide to combine features from several designs, or they may have created personal symbols that they would like to include. After a final plan has been formulated, divide the group into teams of "sketchers, painters, and gluers."

DURING

1. Stretch a long banner-size piece of bulletin board paper on a table.
2. Let participants who have volunteered to sketch out the design do so with pencil.
3. Once the sketching is complete, the banner is ready for paint. Encourage a fairly heavy application of tempera if the group wants the banner to be intense in color.
4. Once the painted areas are dry, other shapes may be glued on. An effective way to increase the contrast and make certain shapes stand out is by outlining them with permanent marker or with oil pastels.
5. Encourage the group to make aesthetic decisions about composition, contrast, and harmony as they work.

AFTER

Hang the banner in an area of the facility that gets a great deal of exposure. Discuss with the group the possibility of finding someone in the community who might be willing to turn the painted banner into a cloth banner. Plan with the group, if they wish, how the participants could make the banner out of fabric. Ask about the possibility of using the banner as a logo for the facility.

ADAPTATION

If there are people in the facility who like to sew, this activity is an opportunity for them to make a contribution to the facility by executing the center design into a banner, quilt, flag, or wall hanging.

Get Up and Go

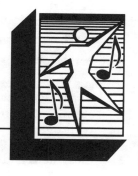

July

| | |

GOALS

- To provide an opportunity for creative expression of feelings
- To increase the daily level of physical activity
- To increase awareness in leisure interests

BEFORE

1. Have participants do the basic warm-up described in the Dance section of Chapter 3.

2. Gather in a circle. Ask participants to introduce themselves and to share one thing they have enjoyed doing during their lives. To spur their memories, first ask the participants to enact such examples as, "rolling out pie crust dough for family dinner," "swimming," "doing the Charleston," "rocking a baby," or "driving to a vacation resort." One way of sequencing the introductions, for those for whom memory loss is not an issue, is to have each person recap the statements of the people who have gone before. The first person begins, then the next person introduces the first person and his or her desire and then introduces himself or herself and his or her secret desire. This continues until everyone has spoken. (If a participant cannot remember a name or desire, assistance should be given.)

DURING

Ask the participants to think about, but not say aloud, a second activity that they have always wanted to do but have never done, and then make up a movement to represent that activity. The other participants should watch and guess what each person wants to do. Ensure that everyone has a chance to participate.

AFTER

Begin a group discussion by asking questions such as:

- What prevents you from doing these activities?
- What equipment do you need to do this activity?
- What can you do to overcome these barriers?
- Who can you contact for assistance?

Encourage the group to spend some time this week thinking about the things that they would like to do but are not doing. Urge the older adults to create realistic dreams and then act on them. Suggest that everyone experiment with one easy to attain goal and take the first step sometime during the next week toward that goal. During another dance activity, allot time for sharing these steps and the results.

ADAPTATION

Persons with developmental disabilities may have trouble forming realistic views of what is possible in the world. During the first part of this lesson, accept fanciful and even outrageous desires from these participants. Ensure that these earnest expressions are met with acceptance. In the "After" section, however, counsel these group members to base their dreams on things that have worked out for them in the past or on activities that they already enjoy doing. The goal that they choose to work on throughout the week should be realistic even if that seems boring to them at the moment. Success in achieving it is then possible.

Going to the Ballet

GOALS

- To increase awareness of cultural opportunities
- To provide an opportunity for socialization and peer interaction
- To provide an opportunity to participate in existing community resources

BEFORE

Tell the group that a trip to see a ballet has been planned. Discounted tickets are often available for senior groups. Sometimes groups can attend a morning rehearsal at little or no cost. The leader should go over with the groups plans for the van, tickets, accommodations, accessibility, and which staff will be there. Begin a group discussion by asking participants such questions as:

- How do you feel about going to a ballet?
- If you have been to a ballet, what was it like? If you have not, what do you think it will be like?
- Where have you seen a ballet before? (Or, where do you suppose ballets are staged?)

If a VCR is available, show a short segment of a video recording of a ballet and have the group discuss how the ballet scene relates to their lives. Using "Swan Lake" as an example, are there "princes" and "evil forces" that seem to be at work in people's lives? How have dances in which the participants have engaged during their lives been similar and/or different from the ballet? Have participants move their arms and/or bodies to express "striving," "indecision," "fear," or "power."

DURING

Take the group to a ballet performance. Remind the group of social skills that should be remembered while at the ballet.

Once the performance begins, the leader should observe the participants' reactions to the performance and make either mental and/or handwritten notes on observed responses. These observations can be discussed with the participants after the performance.

AFTER

On the drive home, the leader can begin a group discussion by asking questions such as:

- What did you enjoy about the performance?
- How did the performance make you feel?
- How did the lighting make you feel?
- What did you think about the costumes?
- Did the movements match the music?
- What do you think the story was about?
- Where else can you go to see a ballet?
- What other kinds of dance do people do?

Encourage participants to read the paper, watch television, and listen to the radio to learn of any dance, art, music, and theater activities that are happening in the community. If they hear of something that they would like to share with the group, suggest that they bring the information to the next meeting. Plan future trips to arts functions.

ADAPTATION

A ballet performance can be a valuable experience for people with visual challenges. The music alone may be sufficiently enjoyable. Consider possible ways to make the event more accessible. For example, binoculars or verbal description during the performance may assist older adults. Also, consider using an audio headset system.

Movement with Props

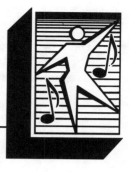

July

MATERIALS

- Sticks
- Butcher paper, construction paper, or fabric
- Markers and paints
- Glue or iron-on adhesive and iron
- Scissors
- Pictures from magazines of typical American activities

BEFORE

Using the materials above, tell the participants to make an American flag and add a personal touch to it. Discuss with the group the meaning of being an American. Were there times in their life when they were glad to be living in America? Once the flag has been made, have each person overlay a magazine picture that represents his or her personal story or special experience with America.

DURING

As a group, do a basic warm-up (see the Dance section of Chapter 3) using the flags as props to help make the movement flow and become larger. Direct the group in making circular, straight, diagonal, and zigzag patterns of different sizes by walking or moving along different pathways. Encourage the participants to come up with ideas of their own. Patriotic or marching music will enhance the activity and set a tone for positive, spontaneous interactions among the participants.

AFTER

Have participants do a basic cool-down. Encourage each of the participants to share their "flag stories" with the group. Continue the discussion by asking questions such as:

- Why do you like living in America? Are there aspects that you do not like?
- What American traditions have you been a part of that you can share with the group?
- What is patriotism?
- In what ways can we be patriotic? Why might it be or not be important to be patriotic? If a person feels that the government is doing something wrong and tries to change it, is he or she being patriotic?

In order to stimulate thoughts or actions about patriotism, suggest that participants look for examples of patriotism in others or act patriotically throughout the week. The next time they gather, allow time to discuss patriotic behavior.

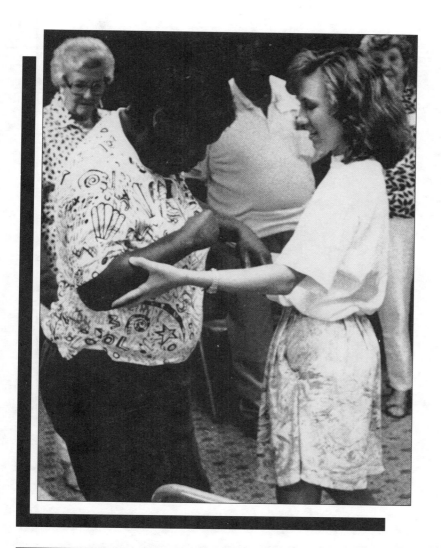

August

Themes:

Summer heat
The beach
Relaxation
Freedom from stress and anxiety

End of Vacation

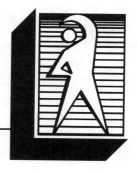

August

GOALS

- To stimulate cognitive functioning by having the group consider vacation pastimes
- To increase muscular strength with the use of light weights
- To improve cardiorespiratory endurance by walking

MATERIALS

- Light weights

BEFORE

Inform the group that as summer comes to an end many people end their vacations and begin doing other things. Ask them to think of things they did while on vacation and what they did when vacation was over.

Warm-up

Mention to participants that some people take trips during vacation.

1. In circle formation, walk in a shuffling manner as if imitating a moving automobile or train.

2. Inhale slowly while raising arms overhead and exhale while lowering arms back to the sides.

3. With hands at shoulder level, palms facing forward, push out with hands while stepping forward on the left foot. Return hands to starting position as the left foot steps back to starting position. Repeat with the right foot.

Stretches

Neck: Mention that some people catch up on sleep and relax during vacation.

1. Ear to shoulder: Tilt head to left (left ear to left shoulder) and hold 10–15 seconds. Tilt head to right (right ear to right shoulder) and hold 10–15 seconds. Repeat 8–10 times.

2. Head drop: Lower chin to chest and hold 10–15 seconds before raising head to starting position. Repeat 8–10 times.

Shoulders/Chest: Mention that people do a variety of exciting things during vacation.

1. Shoulder shrugs: With arms by sides, lift shoulders up toward ears. Hold 10–15 seconds. Repeat 8–10 times.

2. Elbow touches: Standing with feet shoulder-width apart or sitting in a chair, place hands on shoulders and bring elbows together in front of body. Then bring elbows back as far as possible. Repeat 8–10 times.

Arms: Mention that fishing is a favorite vacation pastime for some people.

1. Arm curls: Extend arms down at sides with palms facing forward holding light weights. Bring palms to shoulders and return to starting position. Repeat 8–10 times.

2. Triceps extensions: With right arm bent, hand on shoulder, and elbow pointing toward ceiling, extend the right hand toward the ceiling until the arm is fully extended and slightly forward (as if casting a fishing line). Return to starting position. Repeat 8–10 times. Repeat with the left arm 8–10 times.

3. Wrist circles: Move both hands in clockwise and counter-clockwise circles. Repeat 8–10 times.

Hips/Legs: State that some people walk along the beach and pick up shells on vacation.

1. Half squats: Hold the back of a chair with feet shoulder-width apart. Keep back straight and slowly lower body half way down. Stand back up and repeat 8–10 times.

2. Knee raises: Stand behind a chair and raise the right leg so that the knee is at hip level. Hold 10–15 seconds and return to starting position. Repeat 8–10 times. Repeat with the left leg 8–10 times.

3. Gas pedals: While standing or sitting, extend the right leg forward, point the right foot (extend from the ankle), then turn the right foot back toward the shin (flex at the ankle). Repeat 8–10 times. Repeat with the left leg 8–10 times.

DURING

Tell participants that some people enjoy long walks on their vacations and suggest walking as an activity for the group. Then take the group for a 10- to 15-minute walk. During the walk:

1. Raise both arms in front of the body as high as possible and then lower them.

2. Raise arms overhead and clap both hands.
3. Clap both hands in front of the body.
4. Walk on heels.
5. Walk on toes.
6. Alternate arms while reaching for the sky.
7. Alternate arms while pushing out in front of the body.
8. Raise knees and clap hands while walking.

AFTER

Suggest to the group that people need to settle down when vacation is over, catch their breath from the busy schedule, and get back to routine things.

1. While standing or sitting, slowly bring arms up in front of the body, cross them, and bring them back down again.
2. Shift weight slowly back and forth from one foot to the other.
3. Alternately extend the feet, stretching at the ankle, then relax. (If standing, use the back of a chair for support.)
4. Breathe in and out slowly and feel the body relax.

ADAPTATION

The warm-up may be adapted for persons using wheelchairs by having those whose lower extremities are mobile shuffle in place; if immobile, wheelchairs can be rolled in a circle. If immobility prevents performance of "Knee raises" and "Gas pedals," use the hands and arms rather than feet and legs. The 10- to 15-minute walk can be substituted by a combination of walking in place (if mobility permits) and rolling the wheelchairs in a circle.

Summer Heat

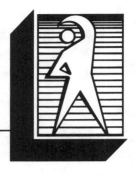

August

GOALS
• To increase muscular strength and endurance with the use of light weights
• To improve aerobic capacity by performing a rhythmical activity
• To explore the effects of heat

MATERIALS

- Light weights
- Cassette player and cassettes

BEFORE

Announce that August is frequently the hottest of the summer months. Mention that although people find ways to cope with the heat, most of us are glad to bid it farewell. Participants can use either no weights, one weight, or two weights in one or both hands—whatever feels comfortable and will give the muscles a workout without excess straining.

Warm-up

Suggest that any activity should be done early in the morning when it is not too hot.

1. Walk in place or around the room, swinging the arms back and forth.
2. Stand in a stationary position and extend the arms overhead, then out to the side, and then down by the thighs.
3. Shift weight from left to right foot, slightly lifting the foot that is not supporting the body's weight.
4. Inhale and exhale slowly as the body stands erect.

Stretch

Neck: State that the heat makes us feel rather droopy.

1. Ear to shoulder: Stand with feet shoulder-width apart and knees slightly bent. Tilt the head to the left (left ear to left shoulder) and hold 10–15 seconds; tilt the head to the right (right ear to right shoulder) and hold 10–15 seconds. Repeat 8–10 times.

2. Chin drop: Lower the chin to the chest and hold for 10–15 seconds before returning to starting position. Repeat 8–10 times.

Shoulders: Suggest that a way to cool off is to go for a swim.

1. Arm strokes: Extend the right arm out in front of the body and press it down by the right side. Repeat with the left arm. Continue alternating strokes 8–10 times.

2. Backward arm circles: Place feet shoulder-width apart and slightly bend knees (or sit in a chair). With arms raised out to the sides at shoulder height and palms facing down, gradually make backward arm circles progressing from small to large. Repeat 8–10 times.

Chest

1. Elbow touches: With feet shoulder-width apart and knees slightly bent (or sitting in a chair), place hands on shoulders and bring elbows together in front of the body. Move elbows back as far as possible. Repeat 8–10 times.

2. Sitting presses: Move arms in front of shoulders with palms facing forward. Push the arms out straight (so that arms are parallel with floor) and return to starting position. Repeat 8–10 times.

Arms: Suggest that the use of fans makes the hot weather tolerable. Hand fans are okay, but ceiling fans are better.

1. Arm curls: Extend arms down at sides with palms facing forward. Hold light weights and bring hands to shoulders; return to starting position and repeat 8–10 times.

2. Triceps extensions: With the right arm bent and the elbow pointed toward the ceiling, extend the right hand toward the ceiling as if turning on a switch. Fully extend the arm, then return to the starting position. Repeat 8–10 times. Repeat with the left arm 8–10 times.

Fingers/Hands: Remind participants that hands get hot and sticky in hot weather.

1. With both hands held in front of the body, touch the thumbs to each of the other fingers on that hand. Repeat 8–10 times.

2. Place hands in front of the body with fingers touching. Stretch fingers apart and hold 10–15 seconds before closing. Repeat 8–10 times.

Torso: Suggest that participants pretend to dive in a pool.

1. Side stretches: Stand with feet shoulder-width apart and knees slightly bent. Slowly lean from the waist toward the left and hold 10–15 seconds.

Lean toward the right side and hold 10–15 seconds. Repeat each side 8–10 times.

2. Forward trunk bends: Stand with knees slightly bent, keeping the head in line with the back. Bend forward and hold 10–15 seconds. Repeat 8–10 times.

Hips/Legs

1. Leg swings: Position body next to a chair for support and carefully swing the right leg forward, then back, then forward again. On every third swing, hold the position momentarily. Repeat 8–10 times. Repeat with the left leg 8–10 times.

2. Heel raises: Stand next to a chair with knees slightly bent. Bend the right knee and raise the left foot off the floor as close as possible to the buttocks. Return to a standing position and repeat with the left leg. Repeat 8–10 times with each leg.

3. Toe raises: Stand behind a chair with knees slightly bent. Raise up onto the balls of both feet, hold and return to starting position. Repeat 8–10 times.

DURING

Lead the group in fitness exercises that use fishing as a theme. Suggested music is "Me and My Shadow."

1. Place fists one on top of the other as if holding a fishing pole. Bring the hands over the right shoulder and "cast" by extending the arms out in front. Repeat 8 times. Repeat to left side 8 times.

2. Practice reeling in something by bending over and straightening from the waist. Repeat 8 times.

3. Cast again, but step out on one foot. Return to standing position. Repeat 8 times, alternating feet.

4. Cast out and reel in, cast out and reel in. Repeat the 4-step sequence 3 times.

Inform the group that the sun is setting, the fish have been caught, and hungry mouths are waiting at home. Walking is the best way to get somewhere when you want to be fit. Suggested music is "Zippidy-Doo-Dah."

1. Step side to side. Repeat 8 times.

2. Walk in place and carefully swing the arms from front to back. Repeat 8 times.

3. Continue walking in place and extend the arms out one at a time as though shaking someone's hand. Repeat 8 times.

4. Walk in place and reach the arms up one at a time. Repeat 8 times.

5. Walk in place, pushing the hands out in front. Repeat 8 times.

6. Return to side to side steps. Repeat 8 times.

7. Continue to step from side-to-side while swaying the arms, too. Repeat 16 times.

8. Finish by swaying from side-to-side and rolling the shoulders. Repeat 8 times.

AFTER

As a final cool-down, lead the group in the following exercises.

1. Slowly roll shoulders backward, one at a time.
2. Slowly roll shoulders forward, one at a time.
3. Interlace fingers and press palms of hands out in front of the body.
4. Extend arms overhead, then stretch out to the sides.

Beach Trip

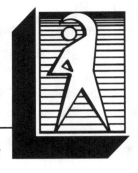

August

GOALS

- To promote the enjoyment of physical activity by relating it to enjoyable summer activities
- To increase muscular strength and endurance with repeated stretching exercises
- To increase the range of joint motion

MATERIALS

- Cassette player and cassettes of music suggesting beach-going
- A collection of big funny beach hats

BEFORE

Suggest that during the month of August people begin to think of the many things they want to do before the summer ends. One of these things it to take another trip to the beach. Encourage the group to imagine that they are at the beach.

Warm-up

Motivate the group to take a short walk as if they were going down to the beach.

1. Walk around the room, or if seated, walk in place, carefully swinging arms back and forth.
2. Perform large circular movements with the arms in front of the body.
3. Inhale and exhale slowly.

Stretch

Neck: Instruct participants to look at the shoreline stretching as far as they can see.

1. Head turns: Turn the head first to the right and then to the left, holding each turn 10–15 seconds. Repeat 8–10 times.

2. Ear to shoulder: Tilt the head to the left (left ear to left shoulder) and hold 10–15 seconds; tilt the head to the right (right ear to right shoulder) and hold 10–15 seconds. Repeat 8–10 times.

Shoulders: Encourage the group to watch the ocean waves roll into the shore and back again.

1. Shoulder circles: Make circles with the shoulders in a forward direction. Repeat 8–10 times. Repeat circles in a backward direction 8–10 times.

2. Arm extensions: Extend arms out to the side at shoulder height, palms facing forward. Bring arms forward until hands touch in front of the body and then return to starting position. Repeat 8–10 times.

Arms: Suggest that participants try their luck fishing off the surf.

1. Back of arms (triceps): With right arm bent and elbow pointed toward the ceiling, extend the right hand toward the ceiling until the arm is fully extended. Return to starting position and repeat with the left arm. Repeat 8–10 times with each arm.

2. Arm curls: Begin with arms extended down by sides, palms facing forward. Bring palms to shoulders, then return to starting position. Repeat 8–10 times.

Hips/Legs: Ask the participants to stoop down and pick up some seashells.

1. Half knee bends: Stand behind a chair and hold the back of it. Place feet shoulder-width apart and bend knees to lower the body half way down. Return to starting position and repeat 8–10 times.

2. Ankle circles: Hold the back of a chair. Extend the right leg forward and turn the right ankle in a circular motion 8–10 times. Repeat with the left leg and ankle.

DURING

Suggest that before they leave the beach, the participants should take a long walk, feeling the sand under their feet, watching the children play with sand buckets, and listening to the ocean as it crashes on the shore.

1. Take participants for a 15-minute walk outdoors (if the weather is cool enough).

2. Assess heart rates at the end of the walk (as shown in the Fitness section in Chapter 3).

An alternate aerobic activity is an imaginary swim in the surf. Suggested music is "By the Sea," or any selection having to do with the ocean.

1. To simulate a swimming stroke, alternate arm reaches and presses.

2. To simulate the backstroke, alternate backward arm circles and "feel the resistance of the water" as the arm comes forward.

3. Alternate backward leg extensions while holding the back of a chair to simulate kicking.

4. Walk in place (as if moving through water and "feeling the water's resistance").

5. Make any other movements that simulate movements in the water.

6. Perform movements that resemble drying off with a towel and getting dressed.

AFTER

Ask group members to think of other things they would like to do before summer ends while they do the following cool-down.

1. Walk in place slowly.

2. Shrug shoulders.

3. Stretch arms overhead.

4. Gently and slowly shake the arms while they hang by the sides.

Fragrances

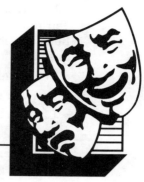

August

GOALS

- To stimulate sensory awareness through smells and fragrances
- To stimulate cognitive functioning
- To increase communication skills

MATERIALS

- Chalkboard or large piece of paper
- Markers or chalk
- Substances with strong smells, such as spices; perfumes; wet petunias; zinnias; kitchen leftovers, such as spaghetti, sauerkraut, or strong-smelling cheese
- Scarves or pieces of fabric to use as blindfolds

BEFORE

Introduce this lesson on senses by explaining how smells are connected with some of our most cherished memories. Begin the group discussion by talking about smells that you remember. Some examples might be Tollhouse chocolate chip cookies baking, a father's pipe, an uncle's barn, cooking sorghum syrup, or the woods after a rain. Then ask group participants what fragrances and aromas they remember. Guide the discussion by eliciting smells from the kitchen, the living room, the outdoors, the barnyard, and so forth. Help each participant to respond. Ask the participants to describe why they remember a particular smell and tell about its origin. Record the responses on a large sheet of paper or on a chalkboard. Encourage group discussion as the participants mention different fragrances.

DURING

1. Divide the group into seated pairs. One person in each pair will be blindfolded while the other will hold up an object to be identified by its smell. Tell the blindfolded participants that they will be asked a series of questions and should tell their answers to their partner. The following is a list of questions for the nonblindfolded partner to ask:

   • Where might you find this odor?

   • Can you remember a specific time when you smelled this odor?

   • Can you remember whom you were with when you smelled this odor?

   Praise the sharing of these experiences.

2. Instruct participants to remove their blindfolds. Ask each pair if they correctly guessed their object.

3. Ask the pairs to switch places. The next person blindfolded should be asked the same series of questions.

4. Instruct the second partner to remove his or her blindfold. Continue the game as time allows with each person being given a different item to smell. If participants are not comfortable being blindfolded, ask them to close their eyes.

AFTER

To extend this lesson into the participants' lives, begin a group discussion by encouraging participants to describe the smells they often smell in their homes or rooms. Help them think of things they might cook that have wonderful aromas, such as homemade candies and baked goods. Encourage brainstorming about ways they might bring aromas into their homes or into the home of a friend to add to the environment's sensory delight.

ADAPTATION

Some older adults' sense of smell is diminished. It is useful to have some very strong odors for them to distinguish. These might include a lit match or cinnamon. Older adults with mental challenges may just name the smell and identify the place where one finds it.

Garden Harvest

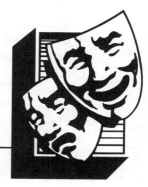

August

GOALS

- To stimulate cognitive functioning
- To have fun
- To increase verbal communication skills
- To increase nonverbal communication skills

MATERIALS

- A few pieces of fruit or vegetables
- Pieces of paper
- Marker or pencil

BEFORE

1. Talk about the joys and hardships of growing a garden. In order for everyone to feel included, ask who has the smallest garden—maybe just a patch of day lilies in the back yard or some plants in the window.

2. Elicit from the participants the names of the tasks involved in making, keeping, and harvesting a garden. One example might be picking squash bugs off the squash vines. As these are named, write each of them on a separate piece of paper.

DURING

1. Distribute the pieces of paper with the names of the chores, giving each participant one to pantomime.

2. Ask each actor to try to perform his or her entire pantomime before the group guesses what is being portrayed. Praise the dramatic ways each actor communicates.

3. If there is time following this activity, a second drama activity can be done. Divide the group into pairs. Each pair will use dialogue and actions to depict growing a garden together, deciding what to plant and where to plant it, hoeing furrows, weeding, dealing with pests, spraying poisons, harvesting the crops, preserving, or canning. Encourage participants to put funny episodes into their skit.

4. Following each skit, lead the group in pointing out the success of the actors in conveying and creating a vivid, fun-filled garden scene.

AFTER

Discuss how gardening activities can be put into practice in the participants' rooms or back yards.

Old Hats, New Ideas

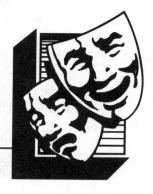

August

MATERIALS

- An assortment of different kinds of hats
- Chalkboard or large piece of paper
- Silk and plastic flowers (optional)
- Bows (optional)
- Hot-melt glue gun (optional)

BEFORE

Discuss with the group how hats often make statements about people's person-alities. For example, a hat may tell something about a person's occupation. Begin a group discussion by asking participants to think of occupations in which special hats or uniforms are required. Record the responses on a large sheet of paper or a chalkboard. Some participants may require help with identi-fying an occupation. Suggestions may include police officer, nurse, doctor, welder, gardener, clown, or firefighter.

DURING

1. Hold up a hat. Begin a group discussion by asking participants what the hat might communicate about the owner's personality or occupation. Such

questions might include whether the owner is neat or sloppy, shy or outgoing, young or old. Participants can also discuss what such a hat's owner would likely be doing during the day. Repeat this kind of discussion with several hats.

2. Begin again with the first hat. Hold it up and, as the leader, do the first pantomime of something such a hat owner might do during the day.

3. Distribute the hats and encourage participants to pantomime what the wearer of each hat might be like.

4. Following the correct identification, the person doing the pantomime can tell why he or she chose that action to go with that hat and, if he or she knows someone like that, to tell about that person.

5. The activity may be repeated with several different hats. Ensure that each person has a chance to discuss his or her pantomime.

6. If possible, cut apart the old hats and reassemble them into fantasy hats, with flowers glued or pinned on. Then ask participants to tell about their fantasy character's personality as seen through the hat. Wire, bobby pins, and a hot-melt glue gun are helpful for attaching objects.

AFTER

Encourage the group to think about their own hats and what these hats tell the world about their personalities and values. As the leader, you should explain first how your personality is shown through your hats. Ideas such as stylish, fashionable, practical, modest, special, hardworking, or not fancy can be sensitively brought out as ways for participants to share their values with their peers. Some participants rarely wear hats in any kind of weather and this "hardiness and strength" can also be discussed. In conclusion, thank the group for their participation in helping to determine how "a hat makes a man or woman."

Another way to extend this lesson is for the participants to make a wild hat at home and wear it for a "Funny Hat Day," with white-elephant type prizes (gag gifts) for such categories as "the wildest, the biggest, or the smallest."

Making Fans for Beating the Heat

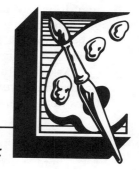

GOALS

- To create handmade fans
- To reminisce about past summer heat experiences
- To discuss the physical dangers of getting overheated
- To plan strategies for keeping cool
- To gain an awareness of fans as an art form

MATERIALS

- Examples of decorated fans (real fans or pictures)
- A variety of paper (11" × 18" heavy white paper, heavy brown paper, and/or wallpaper books)
- Scissors
- Glue
- Hole puncher
- Cord or ribbon
- Large tongue depressors
- Collage materials (e.g., magazines, glitter, paper doilies, fabric scraps)
- Objects for printing
- Liquid acrylic or tempera paint
- Small sponges
- Plastic or styrofoam bowls
- Newspaper
- Chalkboard or large piece of paper
- Chalk or something else with which to write

BEFORE

If possible, bring in a variety of fans or ask participants ahead of time to bring in fans. Books on the history of clothing and fashion, available at local libraries, may illustrate fans as an art form. Stimulate a discussion that will allow the group to share memories of using fans and of hot weather experiences. Ask why it is important not to get overheated. How has the group used fans (in hot weather, a stuffy meeting, or at church)?

Ask the group to reminisce about hot summer days and nights. Perhaps participants would like to put on a skit re-creating such actions and events. Consider writing a list of words about summertime and ways to keep cool.

DURING

1. There are several ways to make decorated fans. Use your own judgment as to what would work best for the particular group. Pages cut from discarded wallpaper pattern books, which are available free of charge from paint stores, make attractive fans. Pictures cut from magazines, parts of paper doilies, and shapes cut from fabric can be glued down carefully onto paper and allowed to dry before the paper is folded into a fan shape. Participants may enjoy printing a pattern on the fan. A variety of objects, such as shells, corks, cut vegetables, paper clips, bottle tops, and so forth, can be pressed into a paint-soaked sponge and then stamped onto the paper to create interesting patterns and designs.

2. Once the fan paper is decorated and dry, fold it every ½" to make an accordion fan.

3. When the fan is folded up, dip the top into glue and then into glitter, then open it up to dry. Little dabs of glue between the folds at the bottom will hold the fan together, or participants may use a paper punch or awl to make a hole in the bottom through which to tie a ribbon or tassel.

4. A holder for the fan can be made by stapling it to a decorated tongue depressor.

AFTER

Stimulate a discussion about the phenomenon of evaporation. Why does high humidity make the body feel hotter? Why do glasses of cold drinks "sweat" on the outside of a glass on a hot day? Make a list on the chalkboard of strategies for keeping cool. For example:

1. Close up the house from early morning until late afternoon.
2. Sit outside on the porch, preferably in a rocker or porch swing.
3. Wet your face and arms with a wet washcloth.
4. Drink cold drinks and use fans.
5. Sleep on the porch.

Another strategy is attitude adjustment. Encourage the group to paint a mental picture of the bad chills and misery of winter (the pain of falls on the ice, cold fingers and feet) and to count their blessings for the hot days.

Clay Castle for Older Adults

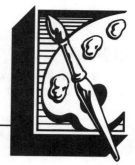

August

GOALS
• To reminisce about beach experiences and making sand castles
• To brainstorm about the perfect facility for older adults
• To create a "castle for older adults" with clay

MATERIALS

- Illustrations of castles (magazine pictures or illustrations of castles in books, especially *Castles* [MacAuley, 1977])
- At least 1 pound of clay per person
- A long piece of bulletin board paper
- Toothpicks
- Plastic knives
- Rolling pins
- Small containers for water
- Cassette player and cassettes (optional)

BEFORE

1. Begin with deep breathing exercises. Encourage participants to relax and imagine that they are sitting on a sandy beach. Have visuals and objects that will provide stimulation. Ocean music also enhances the total experience.

2. Talk about going to the beach—is it a peaceful experience? Ask participants to share memories they have that are associated with the beach.

3. Begin a discussion on sand sculpture. Show illustrations of sand castles. If some of the participants have never been to a beach, focus on imaginary castles.

4. Inquire if the group has ever built "castles in the sky," that is, dreamed about a perfect space for themselves? Invite them to create a perfect castle for older adults. Brainstorm as a group about what sort of rooms it would have. What or who would be inside? Would there be a wall around the castle?

DURING

1. Have everyone sit around a long table covered with bulletin board paper or newspaper and give everyone 1 pound of clay. Inform the group that this clay sculpture will not be fired; at the end of the lesson the clay will be recycled. It is the process of making the dream facility that is valuable, rather than the end product.

2. Suggest that participants make rooms or people for the castle. One good way to create a room is by using the slab method of working with clay. Take a rolling pin and roll the clay out, just like cookie dough. Use a plastic knife to cut out rectangular shapes for walls and floors. Attach shapes at the corners by rubbing with the fingers.

3. Now work on the outside wall for the dream facility. Will it have a turret, a lake, or a pond? Will there be animals or flowers? If so, encourage participants to make these things from clay.

AFTER

Have a group discussion about the dream facility. Is there anything in this imaginary space that might be added to the real facility? What are some improvements in the design of facilities for older adults that would make them more pleasant to be in? Suggest that the participants make a list of things that they would like to see change and give these suggestions to the director.

Creating Summer Note Cards

August

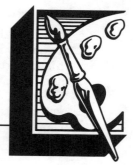

GOALS

- To observe colors and shapes in summer fruit
- To reminisce about summer activities
- To make and send summer greeting cards

MATERIALS

- Images of still life paintings (available from local libraries)
- Variety of summer fruits and vegetables
- Baskets to hold fruit
- Large table cloth
- White paper (should be pre-cut to fit, when folded, into a standard-size envelope)
- Envelopes
- Pencils
- Watercolors
- Brushes
- Containers for water

BEFORE

1. Set up a still life of a variety of summer fruits and vegetables. Watermelons and cantaloupe can be halved to reveal the colorful fruit inside. Squash, cucumbers, eggplant, and zucchini all provide a rich palette of colors and shapes to stimulate visual awareness. Perhaps some of the participants would like to bring in things from their own gardens to add to the composition. A patterned tablecloth or sheet can serve as a backdrop and baskets and containers can add visual interest.

2. Ask the group to share any memories they have associated with the various fruits and vegetables that are in the still life. Are any of the participants gardeners? Ask questions to stimulate reminiscence such as: Where do you remember eating watermelon? Who was with you? What time of day was it? What was the weather like? Did you grow your own melons?

3. Initiate a dialogue with participants about giving friendship. Suggest that it is good to remember friends and rekindle old friendships. One way to do this is through correspondence—making and sending cards. Ask each member of the group to think of someone they would like to reach out to in a friendly, altruistic way. Perhaps a grandchild would appreciate a special note from a grandparent. On the envelope, make a small decoration to make it special.

DURING

1. Hand out white paper, pencils, brushes, and watercolors.

2. Have the group closely observe the still life, looking for lines, shapes, colors, and textures. Hold up one of the vegetables and emphasize the variety of lines and colors within it. Ask participants to focus in on one or two of the fruits and vegetables to use as a design for a greeting card.

3. Tell participants to fold a sheet of heavy 8½" x 11" white drawing paper in half. They may then sketch one or two of the fruits and vegetables on the front of the card. Encourage them to fill the entire space, enlarging the forms to extend to the borders. Incorporate at least one pattern in the design, such as the background.

4. After the pencil sketch is complete, participants are ready to add color. Remind them to really *look* at what they are painting. Is a tomato all one shade of red? What happens to the color near the stem? What will they choose for a background color? Advise them to think of a background color that provides a contrast to objects in the foreground.

AFTER

Find a safe place for the artwork to dry. Participants should have been able to create several cards to send to friends and family. Discuss whom they will correspond with and what they think the reactions will be when their friends and family receive the cards in the mail. Make arrangements for volunteers to help anyone who needs assistance with writing.

Note

Color photocopy one or two of the paintings following each art lesson. Copy black and white drawings. If the center budget allows, color photocopy a few duplicates. Color photocopying costs about 75 cents each; black and white costs about 7 cents each. (Two or four can be done at once. Cut them apart and mount them on folded colored construction paper.) These can be displayed on the art board at the facility. The older adults can photocopy sets of their cards to give, send, display, or sell. It is very reinforcing to have one's work reproduced.

ADAPTATION

For participants with developmental disabilities, it is better to focus on one fruit in the still life. The best fruit for this is the watermelon. Cut a piece of red paper about 8" × 8". Fold the sheet in half, with the crease becoming the "inside" narrow edge of the watermelon wedge. Then cut the outer open sides into a big crescent shape to form the round part of the watermelon slice. Paint a 1-inch green border on the outer edge to represent the rind. The seeds can be made by using real watermelon seeds and gluing them down with white glue, or by using black paint. The seeds can be placed randomly or in rows and columns, or they can be arranged to spell out a person's initials. Open up the card and write the person's name to whom it will be sent, along with a summer greeting and the participant's name as the sender. Before the card is put into an envelope and mailed, it can make an attractive table decoration for a summer watermelon lunch or for a bulletin board display.

The Alphabet: Sign Language

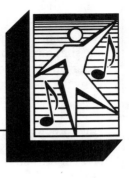

August

GOALS

- To develop skills in sign language
- To enhance communication

MATERIALS

- Any book about basic sign language from a local library. One such book is *Signing Exact English* by Gerilee Gustafson, Donna Pfetzing, and Esther Zawolrow, available from Modern Signs Press, Inc., P.O. Box 1181, Los Alamitos, CA 90720.

BEFORE

Explain to participants that communication can and does occur in a variety of ways that are essential to everyone's well being. Tell them that the eyes and the body can convey a variety of meanings.

Ask participants what signs they use in their daily lives. Have participants pantomime different signs and encourage participants to guess what the different signs mean.

DURING

To teach sign language, begin with numbers because they tend to come naturally. Model a number to the group and then ask them to mirror you. After participants demonstrate knowledge of a few numbers, try signing them in sequence. Once the group has mastered the numbers, start with the alphabet or a few simple phrases in the same manner. It is acceptable if the group learns only a few letters. The point is to enjoy learning, have fun, and participate in what many people call "a ballet with the hands."

AFTER

Ask the participants to sit together in a circle. Begin a group discussion about the importance of signing. Ask questions such as:

- What are some of the ways in which we communicate without talking?
- What would it be like if we could not hear?
- Are there times when it is not appropriate to speak out? How could you use sign language during those times?
- What was it like to learn how to sign?

You may wish to expand the discussion by asking the group where they have seen sign language used in public settings. Examples may include the theater, schools, parks, and places where people meet to socialize.

Creating Patterns from August Movements

August

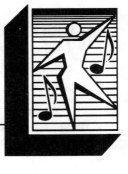

GOALS

- To see how our bodies' movements can be combined to create patterns of beauty
- To use repeated movements to form a dance-like sequence
- To participate as a group to create something more grand than any one individual could create individually

---

MATERIALS

- Any props that can help to simulate the activities, such as pieces of rope to be used to imitate fly fishing casting, sticks to imitate hoes, or ball bats

BEFORE

Discuss the activities done in August. Then, as a group, figure out ways that each of these activites could be conveyed nonverbally through just using our bodies' movements. Create pictures in the participants' minds of what a beautiful pattern would develop if a group of participants all did these movements together, and how the individual differences of each participant would add beauty to the effect.

DURING

Lead the participants in conveying through repeating movements the formation of a dance-like sequence using such motions as swinging in a hammock or a porch swing (two people pretending to rock and one person enacting being rocked), going fishing or to a ball game (and adopting the players' motions as they move in slow motion to swing at balls and catch high flies), hoeing in the garden in unison to the music, or swimming different strokes. Urge participants to carry out the motions slowly and to repeat them in a sequence of four or eight repetitions to make a pattern. After a range of motions have been repeated, have the group repeat the sequence as they become looser and more relaxed and assured of themselves.

AFTER

Discuss how we achieve a sense of gracefulness by imitating these movements in an artistic manner. Talk about how by having others do them with us a pleasing pattern was created. Discuss which of these movements we will do in the hours and days ahead. Have participants think about the way they move and whether their movements are conveying to others the ideas they want them to convey.

Movement Images from Idioms

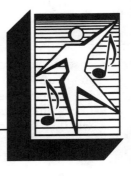

August

GOALS

- To explore the concept of idioms
- To take idioms literally to produce movement images

MATERIALS

- Chalkboard and chalk or paper and markers

BEFORE

Idioms are phrases or expressions whose meanings are different from their literal meanings. Expressions such as "It is over my head" are idioms. Use the chalkboard to create a list of idioms and often-used expressions. Encourage participants to write idioms that they come up with on the chalkboard, or suggest that they select a scribe.

DURING

1. Begin transforming idioms into movement by asking participants to choose an idiom and decide on a way to structure it into an improvisation for one or more participants. Tell them not to share their idea with anyone.

2. Choose one participant to show his or her movement image to the rest of the group without revealing the idiom or expression. Ask the other participants to try to guess what is being represented in movement. For example, the idiom "it is over my head" requires that each participant have a part of his or her body over his or her head at all times.

3. The following are some idioms that are especially good for movement:
   - Armed to the teeth
   - At loose ends

- Bow and scrape
- By leaps and bounds
- Done to a turn
- Down and out
- Down at the mouth
- Draw the line
- Fall head over heels
- Far-reaching effects
- Fast and furious
- Finishing touch
- Firm footing
- Follow in someone's footsteps
- In one fell swoop
- On the spot
- Push comes to shove
- Take it or leave it
- Touch and go

AFTER

Ask participants to sit together in a circle. Begin a group discussion by asking each of the participants questions such as:

- How do you think the idiom that you acted out began?
- How do you feel when you hear an idiom?
- How do you feel when you hear one idiom after another?

Encourage participants to listen for idioms both in their own speech and that of others throughout the week. Suggest that they make up some new idioms for their own use and amusement. They can share these new expressions the next time they meet.

ADAPTATION

Members of the group with developmental disabilities or dementia may have trouble translating idioms into movement. For these members, concentrate on one idiom (e.g., to follow in someone's footsteps). Make sure that everyone has an idea of what the idiom means and how one might use it in everyday language, then turn it into movement. Listen closely to their use of language for idioms and focus on these, as they may be understood more readily.

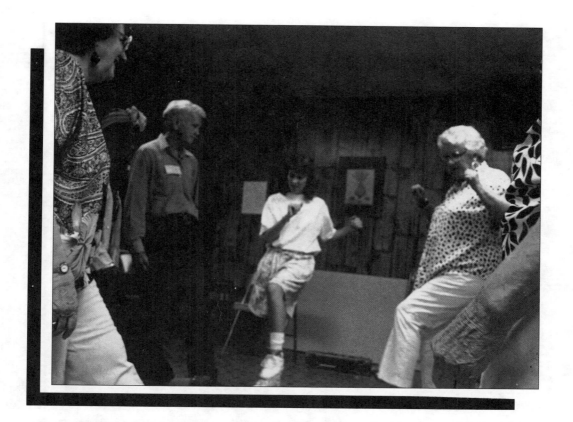

September

Themes:

Back to school
Sports
Learning
Imagination and emotional responsiveness
The dynamic, unfolding spirit of life

Back to School

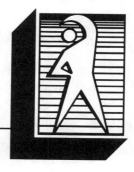

September

GOALS

- To increase muscular strength and endurance with resistance exercises
- To enhance self-esteem by increasing motor skills

MATERIALS

- Cassette player and cassettes

BEFORE

Inform the group that September is the time for students to return to school. Ask them to imagine carrying their school books and walking with their friends. Ask them to remember what it was like on their way to grammar school. Marching music would be appropriate to play during this activity.

Warm-up

1. Stand up or sit up straight and march in place.
2. While marching, swing arms back and forth to loosen them. Continue moving until the end of the first song.
3. Stand in place and bring arms out to the side, like a police officer, to stop traffic. Wave through the people to the left, then the people to the right. Repeat this a few times, then walk across as though escorting people from one curb to the next. As the song comes to an end, slow to a stop and prepare to stretch.

Breathe

1. Step together to form a circle.
2. With feet shoulder-width apart and knees "soft" (slightly bent), roll the pelvis under and relax the arms by the sides.

3. Lift the arms up as high overhead as possible and inhale deeply. Return the arms to the sides and exhale. Repeat 4 times.

Stretch

Standing

1. Stretch arms overhead and stretch the fingers by extending the fingers as wide apart as possible and then as close together as possible. Repeat these finger exercises out to the sides and then close to the body.
2. With arms relaxed by the side of the body, stretch the neck to one side, the other, then down in front.
3. Maintaining good body position, turn the head to see the neighbor to the left, then turn to see the neighbor to the right.
4. While turning the head to one side, exercise the eye muscles by looking as far as possible to that side. Repeat on the other side.

Seated

Ask those who will be doing these exercises while seated to imagine themseves seated in their grammar school classrooms

1. Sit with both feet flat on the floor. To strengthen the abdominal muscles, place the hands on the abdomen and tighten the abdominal muscles. Hold this for 4 counts and release. Repeat 4 times.
2. Place both hands under one thigh and extend the leg forward as far as possible. Feel the stretch in the back of the leg (hamstring). Do not overextend the leg; keep the knee slightly bent. Rotate the ankle 8 times in both directions. Repeat with the other leg.
3. To stretch the arms and legs and work on coordination, extend the left leg and left arm in front and circle the ankle and wrist simultaneously. Repeat with the right arm and leg.
4. Give yourself a hug to loosen the shoulders.

DURING

Continue to work the arms by using resistance. Remember to keep the hands loose (no clenched fists).

1. Extend the arms out to the side with palms facing the ceiling. Touch the hands to the shoulders, then extend the arms. Try to keep the arms at shoulder height. Repeat 8–10 times.
2. Repeat step 1, but turn the palms to the front. Repeat 8–10 times.
3. Repeat step 1, but bring the arms down by the sides with the palms facing the front. Imagine the elbows being pinned to the sides. Repeat 8–10 times.
4. Bring the hands up to the shoulders and press the elbows behind the shoulders. Extend the arms back as far as they can go. This exercises the triceps. Repeat 8–10 times.

Use the resistance exercises while doing the following movements to music.

1. Begin by marching in place with the arms by the sides.
2. Continue to march and extend the arms out to the side. Alternate bringing one hand in and then the other, as with the resistance exercises. Repeat 16 times.
3. Repeat the first four exercises in this "during" section until the music ends.

AFTER

1. Form a circle to do the cool-down.
2. Sway from one side to the other while swinging the arms from side to side.
3. Step forward and backward, bringing the arms front and back.
4. Finish by repeating the three steps in the warm-up.

ADAPTATION

To do these exercises in a seated position, use the hands and arms in lieu of marching with the feet, or march in place. All stretching exercises can be performed in a seated position. If participants are unable to extend their legs, they can extend their arms instead.

Rhythmical activity can be adapted by marching in place in a seated position or marching with hands "slapping" the thighs, or, for a more aerobic exercise, by alternately swinging the bent arms and pointing the fingers to the ears.

At the Ball Game

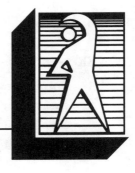

September

GOALS

- To enhance kinesthetic awareness as exercises are performed
- To increase participants' strength with resistance exercises
- To increase strength, endurance, and flexibility by enacting choreographed cheering

---

MATERIALS

- Cassette player and cassettes of school songs

BEFORE

Suggest to the group that any activity is more fun with someone cheering for the participants. Inform the group that in this activity they will cheer their team on to victory. School "fight" songs or chants can be sung or played during the activity.

Warm-up

1. Stand up or sit up straight and march in place.

2. While marching, swing the arms back and forth to loosen them. Try to move together and begin to think like a group of cheerleaders or fans. Continue moving until the end of the first song.

3. Bring the arms out to the side, like a cheerleader. Now bring the arms up into a "V" for victory. Do a small lunge to the left and punch the right hand out in front. Repeat this by lunging out to the right and punching out with the left hand. As the song comes to an end, slow to a stop and prepare to stretch.

Breathe

1. Step together to form a circle.
2. With feet shoulder-width apart and knees "soft" (slightly bent), roll the pelvis under and relax the arms by the sides.
3. Lift the arms up as high overhead as possible and inhale deeply. Return the arms to the sides and exhale. Repeat 4 times.

Stretch

Standing

1. Stretch arms overhead and stretch the fingers by extending the fingers as wide apart as possible and then as close together as possible. Repeat these finger exercises out to the sides and then close to the body.
2. Extend the arms out in front and bring the arms up and down. As the arms move up, flex the hands down, and as the arms move down, flex the hands up. Repeat 8–10 times.
3. With arms relaxed by the side of the body, stretch the neck to one side, the other, then down in front.
4. Maintaining good body position, turn the head to see the neighbor to the left, then turn to see the neighbor to the right.
5. While turning the head to one side, exercise the eye muscles by looking as far as possible to that side. Repeat on the other side.
6. Place the hands on the shoulders and stretch the elbows back as far as possible. If that seems too simple, try placing the hands behind the head and stretching the elbows back as far as possible. Repeat 4 times.

Seated

1. Sit with both feet flat on the floor. To strengthen the abdominal muscles, place the hands on the abdomen and tighten the abdominal muscles. Hold this for 4 counts and release. Repeat 4 times.
2. Place both hands under one thigh and extend the leg as far as possible. Feel the stretch in the back of the leg (hamstring). Do not overextend the leg, keep the knee slightly bent. Rotate the ankle 8 times in both directions. Repeat with the other leg.
3. To stretch the arms and legs and work on coordination, extend the left leg and left arm in front and circle the ankle and wrist simultaneously. Repeat with the right arm and leg.
4. Give yourself a hug to loosen the shoulders.

DURING

Perform the following exercises and develop a few more "cheers" with the group. Remind participants to keep their hands loose when resisting (no clenched fists).

1. Extend the arms out to the side with palms facing the ceiling. Touch the hands to the shoulders, then extend the arms. Try to keep the arms at

shoulder height. Repeat 8–10 times. Alternate touching the shoulder with one arm and then the other. Repeat 8–10 times.

2. Repeat step 1, but turn the palms to the front. Repeat 8–10 times.

3. Repeat step 1, but bring the arms down by the sides with the palms facing the front. Imagine the elbows being pinned to the sides. Repeat 8–10 times.

4. Bring the hands up to the shoulders and press the elbows behind the shoulders. Extend the arms back as far as they can go. This exercises the triceps. Repeat 8–10 times.

5. Place the elbows by the sides and the hands by the shoulders. Extend one arm up as the other stays in place. Alternate lifting one arm up overhead and then the other. Repeat 8–10 times.

Tell the group that they are becoming adept at resistance training. To work on cheering, direct the group to apply some of the arm exercises with the lunges that were used at the beginning. Use some of the movements as participants move to music.

1. Begin by placing the feet apart and hands on hips. Gently sway from side to side. Hold onto a chair if necessary.

2. Lunge left and punch right, return to center, lunge right and punch left, return to center. Repeat these four moves 8 times.

3. Go back to the position in step 1 and sway from left to right 8 times.

4. Repeat the lunges as in step 2, but punch overhead with the opposite arm. Repeat 8–10 times.

5. Go back to the position in step 1 and sway from left to right 8 times.

6. Lunge left and extend the right arm out in front while sweeping the arm across from right to left. Repeat this movement while lunging right, sweeping with the left arm.

7. Go back to the position in step 1 and sway from left to right 8–10 times. Repeat this movement until the end of the song.

AFTER

1. Form a circle to do the cool-down.

2. Sway from one side to the other while swinging the arms from side to side.

3. Step forward and backward, bringing the arms front and back.

4. Drop the arms by the sides and roll the shoulders, first in one direction, then in the other direction.

5. Finish by repeating the three steps used during the warm-up.

6. For a final stretch, give yourself a big hug to stretch the shoulders. Good work, team!

Indian Summer

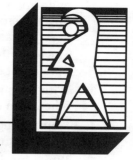

September

MATERIALS

- Cassette player and cassettes of Native American music

BEFORE

Inform the group that September means more hot weather in the south. Announce that in this activity participants will imagine an "Indian summer." Suggested music is "I'm an Indian, Too" from *Annie Get Your Gun.*

Warm-up

1. Stand up or sit up straight and march in place.
2. While marching, move the arms back and forth to loosen them. Try to march together and begin to move like Native Americans moving to the sound of a tom-tom. Continue moving until the end of the first song.
3. Bring the arms out to the side and lift them up to the sky. As the song comes to an end, slow to a stop and prepare to stretch.

Breathe

1. Step together to form a circle.
2. With feet shoulder-width apart and knees "soft" (slightly bent), roll the pelvis under and relax the arms by the sides.
3. Lift the arms up as high overhead as possible and inhale deeply. Return the arms to the sides and exhale. Repeat 4 times.

Stretch

Standing

1. Stretch arms overhead and stretch the fingers by extending the fingers as wide apart as possible and then as close together as possible. Repeat these finger exercises out to the sides and then close to the body.

2. Extend the arms out in front and bring the arms up and down. As the arms move up, flex the hands down, and as the arms move down, flex the hands up. Repeat 8 times.

3. With arms relaxed by the side of the body, stretch the neck to one side, the other, then down in front.

4. Maintaining good body position, turn the head to see the neighbor to the left, then turn to see the neighbor to the right.

5. While turning the head to one side, exercise the eye muscles by looking as far as possible to that side. Repeat on the other side.

6. Place the hands on the shoulders and stretch the elbows back as far as possible. If that seems too simple, try placing the hands behind the head and stretching the elbows back as far as possible. Repeat 4 times.

Seated

1. Sit with both feet flat on the floor. To strengthen the abdominal muscles, place the hands on the abdomen and tighten the abdominal muscles. Hold this for 4 counts and release. Repeat 4 times.

2. Place both hands under one thigh and extend the leg as far as possible. Feel the stretch in the back of the leg (hamstring). Do not overextend the leg, keep the knee slightly bend. Rotate the ankle 8 times in both directions. Repeat with the other leg.

3. To stretch the arms and legs and work on coordination, extend the left leg and left arm in front and circle the ankle and wrist simultaneously. Repeat with the right arm and leg.

4. Give yourself a hug to loosen the shoulders.

DURING

Direct the group to begin this section of the session by performing the following exercises, then suggest the group develop a few more "tribal moves" later. Play music with a slow beat or, if possible, Native American music.

1. Extend the arms out to the side with palms facing the ceiling. Touch the hands to the shoulders, then extend the arms. Try to keep the arms at shoulder height. Repeat 8–10 times. Alternate touching the shoulder with one arm and then the other. Repeat 8–10 times.

2. Repeat step 1, but turn the palms to the front. Repeat 8–10 times.

3. Repeat step 1, but bring the arms down by the sides with the palms facing the front. Imagine the elbows being pinned to the sides. Repeat 8–10 times.

4. Bring the hands up to the shoulders and press the elbows behind the shoulders. Exend the arms back as far as they can go. This exercises the triceps. Repeat 8–10 times.

5. Place the elbows by the sides and the hands by the shoulders. Extend one arm up as the other stays in place. Alternate lifting one arm overhead and then the other. Repeat 8–10 times.

Announce that now the group will combine some of the arm exercises with lunges. Remind participants to pay close attention to posture and center of gravity—stand tall and do not fall.

1. Begin by placing the feet apart and hands on hips. Gently sway from side to side. Hold onto a chair if necessary.
2. Lunge left and punch right, return to center, lunge right and punch left, return to center. Repeat these four moves 8–10 times.
3. Go back to the position in step 1 and sway from left to right 8–10 times.
4. Repeat the lunges as in step 2, but bring the opposite arm all the way around in a circle. Repeat 8–10 times.
5. Go back to the position in step 1 and sway from left to right 8–10 times.
6. Lunge left and extend the right arm out in front while sweeping the arm across from right to left. Repeat this movement while lunging right, sweeping with the left arm.
7. Go back to the position in step 1 and sway from left to right 8–10 times.
8. Now lunge forward on the left foot and sweep both arms forward. Sweep both arms back and return to center. Press down for one count, bending the knees slightly. Repeat the move, lunging on the right foot. Repeat 8–10 times.
9. Continue this last sequence until the end of the song.

AFTER

1. Form a circle to do the cool-down.
2. Sway from one side to the other while carefully swinging the arms from side to side.
3. Step forward and backward, bringing the arms front and back.
4. Drop the arms by the sides and roll the shoulders, first in one direction, then in the other direction.
5. Finish by repeating the lunges, first to the side and then to the center, but this time perform the movements very slowly.
6. For a final stretch, give yourself a big hug to stretch the shoulders.

Food Preferences

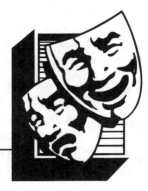

September

MATERIALS

- Chalkboard or large piece of paper
- Chalk or markers

BEFORE

Introduce this activity about foods that people enjoy. Ask the group to name what foods they enjoy. Record the responses on a large sheet of paper or a chalkboard. Begin a group discussion by asking such questions as "Do certain foods remind you of a special place or time? Whom were you with one memorable time when you had that food and what occurred?" Encourage participants to discuss their food selections.

DURING

Role-play preparing favorite foods. Participants might begin, for example, by pantomiming picking blackberries (ouch!), then mixing and rolling out pie dough. The audience can guess what kind of food is being prepared.

AFTER

Discuss memorable actions the actors did in the skits. Discuss if everyone had the same tastes in foods, or if tastes are specific to each person. Encourage participants to remember and tell a story about when they were first exposed to a favorite food. Encourage the group to discuss if differences might depend on where individuals were raised, for example, on farms or in cities. Participants might also discuss whether doctors have made any recommendations to them about such things as fats, sugar, salt, and alcohol.

Solo Pantomimes

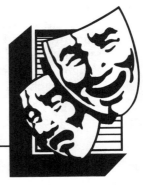

September

MATERIALS

- 3" × 5" index cards
- Pencil or pen

BEFORE

Encourage participants to close their eyes for a minute and think about a chore they can do in their home while sitting down. Seated activities are good to discuss because some participants may use wheelchairs for mobility. Tell participants to open their eyes and begin a group discussion about these chores. Ensure that each participant has a chance to state an activity. Record each response on an index card.

DURING

1. Pass out the index cards that have the name of a daily chore written on them.
2. As the leader, select an index card and do a pantomime to demonstrate the activity to the group.
3. Tell the participants to take a few minutes to think about what they will be doing. Explain that they will pretend to really see the object they are using even though it is not really there.

4. Tell them that if you say the word "freeze," they are to stop moving. When the action is frozen, the audience can brainstorm together to figure out what is going on. Ensure that each participant has a chance to perform.

AFTER

Begin a group discussin by discussing the performances and praising the clever and original things that participants did. Then lead into a discussion of what chores need to be done around one's home or room, and whether one can do the chore oneself or whether someone else should do the chore. Talk about the consequences if the chore remains undone. Also, discuss how one might go about getting started on doing the chore.

ADAPTATION

Assist participants who need help in thinking of an activity by suggesting an activity to them or doing it with them in unison. Another way is to request that a friend work with a challenged individual. Or, show these participants a picture of an activity to act out.

Feels Like...

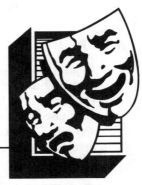

September

GOALS

- To stimulate sensory awareness
- To expand vocabulary
- To think about one's environment
- To promote peer interaction

MATERIALS

- Chalkboard or large piece of paper
- Chalk or markers
- Various objects with different tactile characteristics

BEFORE

1. Introduce this activity about how things feel by talking about the importance of being able to explain the nature of things.

2. Ask participants to name the tactile characteristics of any item that comes to mind. Some participants may require assistance in developing an answer. Record these on a large sheet of paper or chalkboard.

3. Ask the group to name something else that feels each of these ways. Inquire how that characteristic may help the plant, animal, or object in some way.

DURING

1. Divide the group into pairs. One partner will close his or her eyes and the other will take an object. Instruct the participants holding an object to place it in the hands or laps of their partners. Explain that participants with their

eyes shut will describe to their partner what the object "feels" like rather than what it is. Allow adequate time for the pairs to complete this exercise.

2. Tell the pairs to switch roles. Repeat the activity.

AFTER

Assemble the group in a circle. Using the list of tactile characteristics developed earlier, have participants name objects around their homes or rooms that have these characteristics. For example, to the characteristic "noisy," participants might reply vacuum cleaner, microwave oven, cars passing, or factory next door. Discuss whether it is desirable for most things to be soft, smooth, or shiny, or whether some things are more interesting when wrinkled and have a patina of age.

Myth, Art, and Legends of the Pueblos: Creating Clay Storyteller Figures

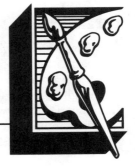

September

MATERIALS

- Map of the United States of America and/or the Four Corners region of the Southwest
- Illustrations or photographs of the artwork and the land of the Pueblo Indians (available in *National Geographic, Arizona Highways,* or other resources that can be found in a local library)
- Illustrations of storyteller figures (available at many local libraries)
- One pound of low-fire clay per person
- Burlap squares
- Toothpicks
- Small sponges
- Containers for water
- Plastic knives

BEFORE

1. Point out the Four Corners region of the Southwest, where major Pueblo settlements exist. Show visuals of the region and the people. Ask partici-

pants to share with the group any trips around the country that they may have taken.

2. Ask the question: "What is a myth or a legend?" Discuss the meaning of myth as both a fascinating story and, on a deeper level, a story that reveals the history and beliefs of a people. Stress the idea that myths often answer important questions or explain things that happen. Some myths have animal characters (e.g., Brer Rabbit, Raven). Some myths are about heroes (e.g., Paul Bunyan, Superman). Many cultures pass these stories down by word of mouth. The storyteller plays an invaluable role in the culture of Native Americans. The Pueblos passed stories down from one generation to the next through storytellers. Usually this was an elder who was greatly revered because of his knowledge of the past.

3. Ask participants if they are storytellers. Do they ever tell their friends and families about things that happened when they were young? Ask them if they would enjoy doing some storytelling at the facility.

4. Show visuals of Pueblo storyteller figures. Incorporate the idea of animals as storytellers.

DURING

Tell participants that they can create their own storyteller from clay. It can be a person or an animal, but there must be a *teller* and a *listener*. Point out the fact that often storyteller figures have their mouths open and appear to be much larger in size than the listener. This exaggeration in scale emphasizes their importance.

Pass out balls of clay, tools, toothpicks, burlap squares, sponges, and water. Demonstrate how to pinch a figure out of a ball of clay. Show methods of attaching parts by dampening the fingers and smoothing two pieces of clay together. Have the group work on individual squares of canvas or burlap. Encourage adding details by drawing in the clay with toothpicks or tools. Place completed sculptures on a shelf to dry.

Note

Fire clay sculptures after they have dried for about 10 days. If the facility does not have access to a kiln, a local potter or art teacher may be able to fire the pieces at no charge.

AFTER

Ask participants to discuss their clay sculptures. How have they exaggerated the size of the storyteller? How have they represented a listener as well as a teller? Have each participant tell the group why he or she chose his or her particular animal or person.

ADAPTATION

September art lessons on myths and legends deal primarily with learning and are intellectually stimulating. Persons with mental challenges might receive benefits from lessons that differ from those done by the rest of the group. Select bold, bright materials and simplify instructions as much as possible.

Creation Myths: Painting Flower Pots

September

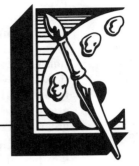

MATERIALS

- Visuals of Southwest Native American pottery (available at a local library)
- Black and white acrylic paint
- Four-inch terra-cotta flower pots (one per person)
- Pencils
- Newsprint
- Water containers
- Small brushes
- Cassette player and blank cassettes (optional)

BEFORE

Review the meaning of myth (discussed in the September art lesson: "Creating Clay Storyteller Figures). Explore the great questions addressed in creation myths. How did the world begin? How did man come into being? Emphasize the role of environment in shaping myths. Many Native American tribes consisted primarily of farmers and their creation myths resulted from their life experiences. They knew that when they planted seeds in the earth new life and growth occurred.

Perhaps participants would like to read or tell their own views of creation, and then as a group discuss similarities and differences between their beliefs. Tape this discussion if possible. It may be more appropriate for people with developmental disabilities to view illustrations of new life (e.g., babies, young animals, seedlings) and discuss the idea of birth and growth in general.

Look at visuals of Southwest Native American decorative pottery. Point out the type of shapes used and how they are repeated to create patterns. Focus on the use of symmetry for balance.

DURING

Pass out pencils, acrylic paintings (black and white), clay flower pots, brushes, and water. Have participants plan their decorative motifs on paper. Encourage them to create a pattern going around the pot or to make a symmetrical design by painting similar shapes on opposite sides of the pot. Suggest that they lightly sketch with a pencil a design on the pot and then paint the shapes with acrylic. Allow the pots to dry.

AFTER

Display the finished pots, discussing how participants created patterns, what shapes they chose and why, and if their container has a symmetrical design. If possible, display the pots in a public place such as in a showcase at a library. Ask group members to bring a small amount of soil to the next class so that they can plant seeds in their new pots.

Note

More information about creation myths can be found in *Myths and Legends of the Indians of the Southwest* (1983) by G. Dutton and C. Olin (Santa Barbara, CA: Bellerphone Books); *Outlines of the Zuni Creation* (1891) by F. Cushing (Washington, DC: Bureau of Ethnology); and *Zuni Folktales* (1901) by F. Cushing (New York: G.P. Putnam and Sons).

Storytelling

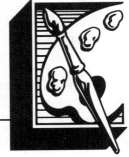

September

GOALS

- To paint clay storyteller figures
- To encourage participants to share life stories and memories
- To foster group interaction through storytelling
- To promote self-awareness and integration through reminiscence

MATERIALS

- Reproduction of a Pueblo storyteller figure (illustrations available at local library)
- Cassette recorder and blank cassettes
- Clay storyteller figures that participants made during the September art lesson: "Creating Clay Storyteller Figures"
- Watercolors
- Brushes
- Containers for water
- Paper and pen

BEFORE

Have participants sit around a long table. Begin the lesson by showing a reproduction of a Pueblo storyteller figure and stressing the importance of older adults as oral historians. Talk about the fact that an older person remembers places and events that are not accessible to young people, and that these memories are valuable and should not be lost—they can connect us to the past. Ask participants to become storytellers and to think of some interesting event in their lives that they would be willing to share with the group. Tape record the session so that participants can hear themselves later.

DURING

Pass out fired clay figures that the group made during the September art lesson: "Creating Clay Storytelling Figures." Also pass out watercolors, brushes, and water. Encourage participants to think about how they want to paint the figures. Will they use realistic colors or will they paint them imaginatively? Perhaps some people will want to leave their figures the color of the clay. Tell participants to use their own aesthetic judgment with their designs. While participants are painting their figures they can also tell their stories.

AFTER

Transcribe each participant's story, if possible, and give it back to him or her. The clay sculptures can be put on display along with the written stories.

Building a Phrase

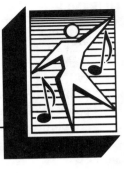

September

GOALS

- To build a phrase movement and make a story from it
- To move and converse

BEFORE

Have participants sit in a circle of chairs. Begin group stories by asking one person to create an opening sentence and each of the other participants to contribute a sentence that advances the story. The story should conclude by the time it returns to the first participant. Ensure that each person has an opportunity to begin a story.

DURING

1. Invite the group to build "movement stories." Have a volunteer give one movement, then ask another person for another movement. Build a phrase: 1, 1-2, 1-2-3, 1-2-3-4, and so forth. It would be best not to exceed eight movements.

2. Once the group has the pattern down (counting out loud may help), ask the group how they would like to perform it. Examples include fast and slow movement, small and large movement, quiet and loud movement. Let the group come up with ideas.

3. Once this has been explored, create another "movement story."

4. When the group is ready, combine the two forms of storytelling by asking a participant to create both a sentence and a movement and have every person build upon the tale.

AFTER

Have the participants discuss the similarities between the dances they created and the stories. Questioning should center on the following topics:

- How it felt to create a dance as a group
- How it felt to create a group story and whether it turned out as expected
- Listing activities that people and animals do in groups (Answers might include potluck dinners, the building of houses, quiltmaking, the damming of rivers by beavers, the building of nests by birds.)
- Other activities the participants can do in groups
- Discussing the pros and cons of working in a group

Suggest that throughout the week participants find at least one thing that they usually do alone, but could do with someone else. Perhaps a chore could be shared, such as shopping—share coupons, carpool, carry bags together, and exchange shopping tips. Perhaps a decision that one would normally make alone could be brought to another's attention and his or her advice could be obtained. From the activities that the older adults mention that they have done or could do with someone else, consider planning future group activities together.

Trust Walks

September

MATERIALS

- One blindfold for each pair of participants

BEFORE

Ask the participants to divide into pairs. Let them get comfortable walking around the room together. Tell them they need to stay together. They may hold hands or walk arm in arm if they wish. Have them take turns, momentarily closing their eyes and feeling surfaces. This is to prepare them for the experience of walking together when one of them is blindfolded.

DURING

Give one partner in every pair a blindfold. Tell the other partner to lead the "blind" partner around the room. Partners should not talk. Tell the leader of each pair to walk very slowly and to be sure to give clear directions with their bodies to their blindfolded partners so that they may follow them with confidence. Instruct the leaders to give the blindfolded partners as many sensory experiences as they can find in the room. They can put their partners' hands on surfaces so they feel them, they can expose them to different sounds or smells, they can position them so that they feel a cool breeeze or a heater, they can lead them into a lighter or darker area, and so forth. Instruct the participants wearing blindfolds to keep all of their senses open. The leaders are responsible for the safety of their blindfolded partners and should be sure not to lead them into furniture or into other people. After about 5–10 minutes, let the "blind" partners take off their blindfolds and let the partners share experiences. Then let the "blind" partners become the leaders.

AFTER

When both partners have experienced leading and following, ask the group to come together in a circle and share their experiences. What different sense experiences did people have? Which senses did they notice more without their sight? What was it like to perceive the room with all senses except sight? What new things did they notice? How did it feel being led in this way? Were the "blind" able to trust those leading them? What did leaders do that made their partners comfortable following them?

Encourage participants to explore their living quarters in similar manners. Perhaps a friend could watch just in case something unexpected happens. If blind exploration is too involved, suggest that participants find moments to shut their eyes and just listen.

Breath Affects Movement

September

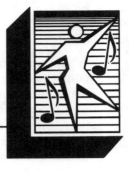

MATERIALS

- Well in advance of the lesson, encourage participants to explore their surroundings for the effects of wind. Ask them to bring pictures, photographs that they have taken, sketches that they have made, and stories that they have heard about wind.
- An illustration of Botticelli's "The Birth of Venus" (or other pictures in which wind appears human-like)

BEFORE

Assemble the group around a table or in some other position that is good for sharing photographs, illustrations, and stories. Invite the participants to share the pictures, drawings, and stories that they brought about the effect of wind. Show the group a picture of wind made to appear human to introduce the idea that today they are going to "become" wind.

DURING

Divide the group into halves. One side will be the wind and the other side will show the effects of wind. Give the wind group different types of wind to embody: warm, gentle wind; cold, sneaky wind; happy, gusty wind; or mean, stormy wind. Encourage this group to actually make the sound of wind while moving their bodies like the kind of wind they are depicting. Tell this group to restrict their movement to only one small area.

The group that is affected by the wind is allowed to move around the room as freely as they like. Ask this group to pretend to be blown by the wind and to express the emotion that they associate with being blown by a certain kind of wind. After the groups have had ample time to experience their parts, tell the groups to switch roles.

AFTER

Instruct participants to sit in comfortable positions. Discuss some ideas about breath. Breathing is one of the most basic things that we do. By breathing slowly and evenly, we can relax. Suggest that participants place their hands on their abdominal region so they can ensure that they are breathing from the diaphragm and not from the upper chest only. Challenge the group to think only about their breathing and not about anything else. If they do find themselves thinking about other things, ask them to return their thoughts to their breathing.

Ask the group to come together in a circle. Begin a group discussion by asking:

- What did it feel like when you were breathing deeply?
- Do you think it feels differently to breathe indoors than to breathe outdoors?
- How do changes in temperature affect what it feels like when you breathe?
- Why is breathing so important?

If participants felt that concentrating on breathing was relaxing, suggest that throughout the week they remain aware of their own breathing and that they take time out to just concentrate on breathing.

ADAPTATION

When involved in the part of the activity in which one group blows like the wind and the other group responds to the wind, warn members of the group who have trouble maintaining balance not to get carried away with the drama of the activity or be "blown over" by the wind, as this might cause real injury. Instead, suggest that the entire group respond as if they were taking part in a slow-motion film.

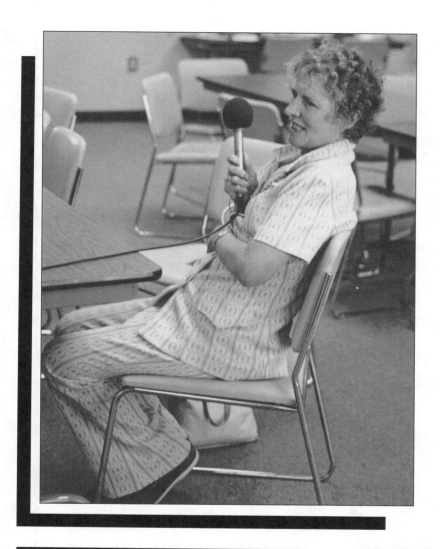

October

Themes:

Halloween
Autumn
Aroused feelings and passions
Revitalization
Enthusiasm
Life enhancement

Costume Party

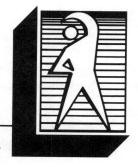

October

GOALS

- To increase range of motion by performing stretching exercises
- To increase aerobic activity with sustained walking
- To integrate physical activity with the celebration of Halloween
- To promote enjoyment of physical activity

MATERIALS

- Light scarves (optional)

BEFORE

Ask the group to think about Halloween and some of the ways they have celebrated it in the past. Ask them to imagine that they have been invited to serve as judges at a Halloween costume party. Inform them that their task will be to determine the best costume as the characters parade past.

DURING

Warm-up

Suggest that before participants take their seats on the judge's stand, they mingle with the crowd to get a good view.

1. Begin with weight equally distributed on both feet.
2. Towel step: Lightly touch the ball of the right foot to the front, then return the foot to center, then touch the ball of the left foot to the front, then return to center. Swing arms in scissor movement in opposition to foot pattern. Repeat several times.

3. Walk in single file around the room, swinging the arms back and forth. Return to original position.

4. With hands on hips, breathe in and out slowly and deeply several times.

Stretch

Announce that the group is ready to begin judging duties and that the contestants are lining up to begin their march.

Neck: Tell participants to watch closely to see who will come by first, then check their score cards to see that they are in order.

1. Look left/look right: Turn the head to the left and hold 10 seconds; turn the head to the right and hold 10 seconds. Repeat 8–10 times.

2. Look up/look down: Look straight ahead, then lower chin to chest and hold for 10 seconds. Repeat 8–10 times.

Shoulders: Announce that the first contestant is dressed as a black cat. Watch his back curl and note his slinky movements.

1. Shoulder shrugs: Raise the shoulders up toward the ears and hold 10 seconds. Repeat 8–10 times.

2. Alternate shoulder circles: Move the right shoulder in a circular, backward motion several times. Repeat the movement using the left shoulder.

Chest: The next contestant seems to be a goblin of sorts (rather spooky). Others are shying away.

1. Elbow touches: With feet shoulder-width apart and knees slightly bent, place both hands on the shoulders and bring the elbows together in front of the body, then move arms back as far as possible. Repeat 8–10 times.

2. Arm presses: With elbows bent and hands at shoulders with palms facing forward, push arms straight out (parallel to the floor), then return to starting position. Repeat 8–10 times.

Arms: (Scarves may be used to add to the flowing motion of the arm swings.) Narrate that a ghost arrives next and ask the group to watch the graceful, flowing movement she makes as she goes by.

1. Scissor arm swings: Standing with feet a comfortable distance apart, swing one arm forward and the other back while slightly and rhythmically bending the knees. Repeat 8–10 times.

2. Double arm swings: Begin with hands and arms in front of the body and swing both arms in a clockwise direction. Repeat in the opposite direction. Repeat 8–10 times.

3. Arm curls: With arms by sides, palms facing forward, bend elbows and bring palms to the shoulders. Return to starting position. Repeat 8–10 times.

Fingers/Hands: Announce that someone dressed as a witch walks by with hands outstretched, casting her spell.

1. Finger presses: Hold hands out, palms down. Begin with the little fingers on each hand and press down with each finger as if casting a spell.

2. Finger stretches: Make fists with both hands in front of the body, then spread and straighten the fingers. Repeat 8–10 times, alternately making fists and extending fingers.

Hips/Legs: Announce that someone in a skeleton costume is ready for judging.

1. Knee raises: Stand behind a chair for support and raise the right leg, bringing the knee toward the chest. Return to starting position and repeat with the left leg. Repeat 8–10 times.

2. Half squats: Stand beside a chair for support, place feet shoulder-width apart, bend knees, then slowly lower the body halfway down. Raise body up. Repeat 8–10 times.

3. Reverse leg raises: With body positioned next to a chair, raise extended outside leg backward 6–12 inches from the floor.

Accompany the group on a 15-minute walk. Along the way encourage them to discuss Halloween costumes. At the end of the walk, instruct the group to assess their heart rates (as shown in the Fitness section in Chapter 3).

AFTER

Ask group members to think about which of the imaginary contestants they would have selected as having the best costume while they cool down.

1. Slowly walk around the room, forming a big circle.

2. Alternately stretch each arm overhead. Repeat 8–10 times.

3. Bend knees slightly and swing arms back, straighten legs and swing arms forward. Repeat 8–10 times.

4. Inhale and exhale slowly.

ADAPTATION

All of the warm-up and stretching exercises may be performed by persons in wheelchairs with the exception of half squats and reverse leg raises. Lower leg lifts may be substituted for these exercises if mobility in lower extremities permits.

Sights, Sounds, and Smells of Autumn

October

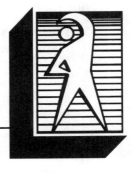

GOALS

- To increase the awareness of the sights, sounds, and smells of autumn
- To promote muscular strength and endurance with the use of light weights
- To increase range of joint motion
- To improve balance

MATERIALS

- Beanbags or other light weights, such as 16 oz. cans of food

BEFORE

Ask the group to think of the crisp, cool air of early October, the leaves changing colors and falling from the trees, and the smell of logs burning in fireplaces.

Warm-up

Suggest that there is something about autumn that makes people feel energetic.

1. Form a big circle and walk briskly around the room, swinging the arms back and forth. (If space is limited, walk in place.)

2. With hands at sides, inhale and raise arms out to the sides; exhale and lower arms to the starting position.

3. While standing, lift right leg forward and carefully kick across the body toward the left. Alternate legs.

Stretch

Neck: Announce that during autumn the leaves turn to red, brown, and gold almost before one's eyes.

1. Look left/look right: Turn the head to the left and hold 10 seconds; turn the head to the right and hold 10 seconds. Repeat 8–10 times.
2. Ear to shoulder: Tilt the head to the left (left ear to left shoulder) and hold 10 seconds; tilt the head to the right (right ear to right shoulder) and hold 10 seconds. Repeat 8–10 times.

Shoulders: Tell participants that the cool air brings a chill to the body. It is time to get out warm sweaters.

1. Shoulder shrugs: Raise the shoulders up toward the ears and hold 10 seconds. Repeat 8–10 times.
2. Zipper stretches: Place the right arm over the right shoulder, then bring the left arm up the back as far as possible and attempt to grasp both hands together.

Chest: (use improvised weights)

1. Elbow touches: With feet shoulder-width apart and knees slightly bent, place both hands on the shoulders and bring the elbows together in front of the body, then move arms back as far as possible. Repeat 8–10 times.
2. Arm presses: With elbows bent and hands at shoulders with palms facing forward, push arms straight out (parallel to the floor), then return to starting position. Repeat 8–10 times.

Arms

1. Arm curls: With arms by sides, palms facing forward, bend elbows and raise arms so palms touch the shoulders. Return to starting position. Repeat 8–10 times.
2. Triceps extensions: With the right arm bent and the right elbow pointed toward the ceiling, extend the right hand toward the ceiling until the arm is fully extended. Return to starting position and repeat with the left arm. Repeat with each arm 8–10 times.

Torso

1. Side stretches: Standing with feet shoulder-width apart and knees slightly bent, slowly lean from the waist toward the left and hold 10 seconds. After returning to an upright position, repeat to the right side. Continue alternating left and right 10 times.
2. Knee touches: Standing next to a chair for support, place the left hand on the left shoulder. Raise the right leg to hip level and touch the right knee with the left elbow. Return to starting position and alternate sides. Repeat 8–10 times.

Hips/Legs: Suggest that the group imagine the sound of leaves being kicked and crushed as they walk.

1. Front leg raises: Stand next to a chair with the left hand on the chair for support, bend knees slightly, then raise the right leg forward up to hip level. Return to starting position. Repeat 8–10 times with each leg.

2. Half squats: Stand behind a chair for support, place feet shoulder-width apart, bend knees, then lower the body halfway down. Raise body up. Repeat 8–10 times.

3. Heel kicks: Stand behind a chair for support, bend the right knee and raise the right foot up as close as possible to the buttocks. Return to starting position and switch legs. Repeat 8–10 times, alternating legs.

4. Toe raises: Stand behind a chair for support, slightly bend knees, then transfer weight to balls of feet. Hold for 10 seconds then return to starting position. Repeat 8–10 times.

DURING

Advise the group that going for a walk is nice almost anytime, but it is particularly nice in autumn, when the leaves have turned a rich yellow, orange, and brown. Perhaps a nearby tree has turned flame red or bright yellow.

Ask participants to take a short walk outdoors to see this special autumn sight and also to note other special autumn changes seen in nature. (If the weather does not allow for a walk outdoors, walk within the facility.) Encourage participants to point out the various visible indications of autumn during the walk. Participants who use walkers or wheelchairs might go on a shorter walk outdoors, noting the feeling of the breeze and the autumn smells and sights. Upon completion of the walk, instruct the group to assess their heart rates, as discussed in the Fitness section in Chapter 3.

AFTER

Have the group close their eyes and imagine all the sights and smells of autumn. Ask them to open their eyes and participate in the following cool-down.

1. Walk in place slowly.

2. Bring arms straight out in front of the body, then out to the sides, then back to starting position.

3. Continue walking alternately pushing the arms out in front of the body.

4. Raise the right knee and clap hands beneath the right thigh. Raise the left knee and clap hands beneath the left thigh. Alternate legs 8 times.

5. With body positioned next to a chair for support, place weight on the right foot and lift the left foot slightly off the floor. Repeat with weight on the left foot. Continue alternating legs, holding each position 10 seconds. Repeat 8 times.

6. Bring arms up and out to the sides, cross arms in front of the body, and give yourself a big hug.

Trick or Treat

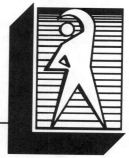

October

MATERIALS

- Square dance music and cassette player

BEFORE

Talk with the group about the origin of Halloween. Ask them what comes to their minds when they think of Halloween.

Warm-up

Suggest that one does not have to be a youngster to enjoy playing trick-or-treat.

1. Walk briskly in place, swinging arms back and forth for 1½–2 minutes.

2. With feet a comfortable distance apart, alternately circle arms from front to back, completing each circle with one arm before the other arm moves. Repeat 4–6 times.

3. With feet shoulder-width apart and knees slightly bent, lean to the right from the waist and hold 5 seconds, then lean to the left for 5 seconds. Repeat 3–4 times.

4. With hands on hips, inhale slowly and deeply, then exhale.

Stretch

Neck: Tell the group that sometimes a look and a smile is a treat.

1. Look down/look up: Look straight ahead, then lower chin to chest and hold for 10 seconds. Repeat 8–10 times.

2. Look right/look left: Turn the head to the left and hold 10 seconds; turn head to the right and hold 10 seconds. Repeat 8–10 times.

Shoulders/Arms: Suggest to the group that instead of fruit and candy, a picture of themselves might be a real treat for someone.

1. Picture frame stretches: Place left hand on right elbow and right hand on left elbow, then raise arms above head. Hold 10–15 seconds. Repeat 8–10 times.

2. Arm stretches: With arms by sides, palms facing outward, bring hands as high above head as possible. Return to starting position. Repeat 8–10 times.

3. Arm curls: With arms by sides, palms facing forward, bend elbows and bring palms to the shoulders. Return to starting position. Repeat 8–10 times.

Torso

1. Side bends: Stand next to a chair for support with feet shoulder-width apart, then slowly lean to the right by sliding the right fingertips down the right thigh. Switch sides. Repeat 8–10 times.

2. Half turns: With arms extended out to sides, slowly turn body one-quarter turn to the right, then back to the original position, then one-quarter turn to the left. Repeat 8–10 times.

Hips/Legs

1. Front leg raises: Stand next to a chair with the left hand on the chair for support, bend knees slightly, then raise the right leg forward up to hip level. Return to starting position. Repeat 8–10 times with each leg.

2. Crossovers: Standing behind a chair for support, carefully swing the extended right leg across the body toward the left and return to starting position. Switch legs. Repeat 8–10 times.

3. Heel kicks: Stand behind a chair for support, bend the right knee and raise the right foot up as close as possible to the buttocks. Return to starting position and switch legs. Repeat 8–10 times, alternating legs.

Ankles/Feet: Ankles and feet also benefit from exercise. Announce that at the end of a busy day just propping the feet up and relaxing is a treat.

1. Ankle circles: Stand next to a chair for support, extend the outside leg, and turn the ankle in a circular motion. Change directions. Repeat with the other ankle.

2. Toe/arch flexibility: Stand next to a chair for support, extend the right foot, and curl the toes under. Repeat with the left foot. Repeat 8–10 times with each foot.

DURING

As a special treat for the group, invite someone who square dances or calls square dances to come in and teach or lead the group in a few simple dances. Assess participants' heart rates after the dance.

AFTER

Ask the group to form a circle and share some of their Halloween memories while they do cool-down exercises.

1. Ask the group to form a circle and face inward.
2. Perform alternate shoulder circles backward, then forward.
3. Alternately stretch right and left arms overhead.
4. Bend forward and extend both arms straight in front of the body. Raise arms overhead and straighten back. Slowly lower arms to sides.

Fall Playwriting

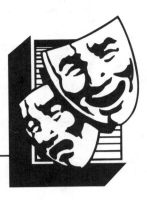

October

MATERIALS

- Sheets of paper
- Pens or pencils

BEFORE

Masks and other coverings on our heads have an effect of letting us be transformed into other characters, and we can then move and dance like these new characters.

Whatever supplies are available (yarn, cotton balls, paper scraps, or markers) will dictate how the mask is made. Be sure to cut out large holes for the eyes, and encourage freedom of movement as participants put on the masks and do movement activities.

Discuss what special things are done more during October than during any other month. Write each of these activities on separate sheets of paper. For example, decorative arrangements of fall leaves are made, decorative gourds are shellacked or waxed, pumpkins are carved and set out on porches, and football games are watched on television. Also, late crops, such as winter squash, tomatoes, potatoes, and apples, may be brought in and stored. Often, walks or rides are taken to view the changing colors of fall. Perhaps participants have baked certain special foods at this time, such as sweet potato pie or pecan pie.

DURING

1. Encourage participants to plan an October skit that incorporates as many seasonally appropriate things as they can fit into it. Divide the participants into groups of 4–5 to plan their October skit. It may be funny, silly, or realistic.

2. Distribute the sheets of paper with October activities written on them. These will provide each group with different activities to incorporate in their skit. Encourage each group to liven up their skit with action (for example, raking leaves, gardening, playing football).

3. Allow adequate time for each group to prepare, then ask each group to perform their skit.

AFTER

After each skit, encourage the audience to talk about it. Help the group to point out the special dramatic devices the actors used. For example, one character may have spoken in a shrill voice or someone may have portrayed a little girl with a whining voice. Discuss how the actors portrayed their characters' personalities. Describe whether each actor's character had the same personality or a different personality from the actor's true personality. Encourage the actor to talk about this "other personality," and whether it was a memory of someone from the past or present. Solicit from the audience members the memories that each skit brought to their minds.

Storytelling

October

MATERIALS

- Chalkboard and chalk or large piece of paper and marker
- Halloween props, such as witches' hats (optional)

BEFORE

Introduce October as a month of magic, mystery, folk tales, superstitions, and ghost stories. Explain that in this activity each group will make up a Halloween story. Make a list of the participants' ideas about Halloween story characters and plot situations. Discuss how Halloween stories usually build up suspense by repetition.

DURING

1. Divide the participants into groups of four or five. Explain that they will create a Halloween story to present to the group. It may be scary, funny, silly, or realistic. It may be about how children in costume go from door to door, for example. Allow adequate time for each group to prepare their presentation.

2. Ask each group to perform their skit. After each skit, encourage the group to talk about the plot, how the characters were portrayed, and what

prompted them to do that particular skit. Help them to point out the dramatic devices the actors used (e.g., "a deep, wobbly voice").

AFTER

Discuss what purpose Halloween serves in our society. Encourage brainstorming about how the participants could participate in celebrating Halloween outside the immediate group. For example, discuss the feasibility of having a Halloween party for the neighborhood children, with the youngsters doing skits for the older adults and vice versa.

ADAPTATION

Some participants, including those with mental challenge, may not like the idea of scary stories. An age-appropriate way to approach the idea of Halloween is role-playing greeting children who come to the door trick-or-treating. Alternatively, participants can take turns acting as householders or acting as the different nonfrightening characters, such as princesses and superheroes.

Hosting a Holiday Party

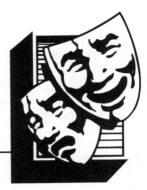

October

GOALS

- To provide an opportunity to plan a special event
- To increase group interaction skills

MATERIALS

- Chalkboard and chalk or large piece of paper and marker

BEFORE

1. Discuss reasons why people like to give parties (e.g., they have something special to show off, a happy event to celebrate, or they want to get together with friends). Encourage participants to plan and carry out a special Halloween party for others. The invitees could be other residents of the facility or they could come from another location, such as a home for youth in trouble, a nearby care facility, or a school.

2. Participants should divide up into four groups to plan the party. Help each participant decide which group he or she would like to join. The first group can make a list of guests, make invitations, and make arrangements for the guests to get to the party. The second group can decide on the entertainment for the party—games, skits from the October drama activity "Storytelling" could be presented, a haunted room, music to play and songs to sing. The third group can be in charge of refreshments and decide what refreshments will be served. They can contact local businesses to have the refreshments donated. The fourth group can be in charge of the set-up and decorations. Explain that the goal of each group will be to get as many things donated as possible and to make whatever else is needed.

3. Allow adequate time for the groups to meet and begin to discuss their plans. Record the group assignments on a large sheet of paper or a chalkboard.

DURING

It may be useful to have a dress rehearsal for the party a day before the actual event. Discuss whether there needs to be more or less entertainment and how the decorations can be enhanced. Give every participant one or two duties to perform when the guests arrive. Everyone should help the guests have a good time. Praise the participants for their roles in carrying out the party.

AFTER

After the party is over and the guests have left, have each group report on how its role in the party went. Congratulate the groups on their planning. Point out how the success of the party depended on the ability of everyone to work together. Discuss if they learned anything from having this party. Perhaps certain participants demonstrated abilities of which the group was previously unaware.

Receiving Positive Messages (Part 1)

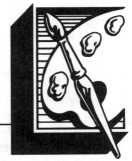

October

GOALS

- To have participants give and receive positive messages
- To promote self-esteem through positive feedback
- To create clay containers to hold messages

MATERIALS

- Two pounds of low-fire clay per person
- Rolling pins or heavy cardboard tubes
- ¼" lattice strips cut 12" in length (at least 2 pairs per participant)
- Burlap squares
- Plastic knives
- Containers for water
- Small sponges
- Natural objects to press into clay
- Toothpicks
- Sheets of scrap paper for use as a pattern
- Decorative boxes, such as hat boxes, gift boxes, wooden boxes, or china boxes

BEFORE

Introduce the season of Halloween by focusing on the theme of giving positive messages as treats instead of candy. Halloween is usually thought of as a time to trick-or-treat. Because these tricks or treats are traditionally received in a bag or container of some kind, tell the group that they will make a clay container. Then they will give each other treats—positive messages about each other—to go in them. Ask participants to look at the variety of sizes and shapes as well as decorative motifs on the different boxes brought to class.

DURING

1. Participants need to roll out five slabs of clay to create a small box. Two pairs of slabs that are the same size and one slab for the bottom of the container that is the width of the sides must be made. It would be helpful to cut out paper patterns for the sides and bottom of the container to use as patterns.

2. Demonstrate rolling out slabs of clay. Press down gently on a ball of clay about the size of a large orange. Place flattened ball between two strips of ¼" lattice. With a rolling pin (or heavy cardboard tube), continue rolling the clay until it has reached the desired size. Place paper pattern on clay slab and trim away excess with plastic knife. Continue rolling until all five slabs have been made.

3. Before attaching sides to the bottom of the container, encourage participants to add texture and patterns by pressing objects into the clay or by drawing into it carefully with toothpicks. After they have added decorative elements, they are ready to attach the slabs by carefully moistening the edges of the clay and smoothing them with their fingers.

4. Ask the group if anyone would like to make a lid for his or her container. If so, this is an opportunity to be really creative! Roll out another slab of clay and, using the paper pattern for the bottom of the container, cut the lid out a fraction larger than the bottom so that is will fit over the sides of the box. An interesting handle can be formed and added. This could be as simple as a strip of clay or as complex as an animal or a flower.

AFTER

Once the clay boxes are complete, put them in a safe place to dry. After about 10 days they should be ready to fire. Ask participants to be thinking about positive messages they would like to make for themselves and each other to go in the containers. Suggest that during the next 2 weeks they keep a notebook to write down affirmations for their friends at the facility or affirmations about themselves.

ADAPTATION

For participants with developmental disabilities or dementia, leave out the suggestion that during the next 2 weeks they keep a notebook to write down affirmations for their friends or themselves. If making the clay box is too difficult for persons with mental challenges, ask them to paint or glue patterned paper to an already existing box with a lid. Instead of glazing or painting, they can coat the entire box with an acrylic coating.

Receiving Positive Messages (Part 2)

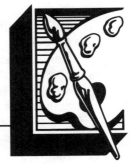

October

GOALS

- To have participants give and receive positive messages
- To decorate clay boxes created in the October art lesson: "Receiving Positive Messages (Part 1)"

MATERIALS

- Acrylic paints
- Brushes
- Containers for water
- Pre-cut pieces of construction paper (cut each sheet into eight pieces)
- Pencils or pens
- Fired clay boxes from October art lesson: "Receiving Positive Messages (Part 1)"
- A variety of decorative containers for display

BEFORE

1. Have participants sit in a circle. Ask participants to get out the notebooks they started after the October art lesson, "Receiving Positive Messages (Part 1)" and to think about the positive messages written about friends at the facility.

2. Pass out to each person several pre-cut pieces of construction paper and something with which to write. Ask them to write one affirmation (or they can draw a symbol if they cannot write) on each piece of paper to give each person in the group. These positive messages will be put in the special clay container that the group is going to decorate.

DURING

1. Point out the variety of decorative containers or displays. Discuss the use of color, shapes, lines, and patterns that are a part of each design.

2. Pass out the participants' clay boxes, paints, brushes, and water. Tell the participants to plan their own unique designs. Do they want to paint the entire box one color or a variety of colors? Will they add patterns after the initial coat of paint is dry or will they paint on patterns and let part of the natural color of the clay show through?

3. Encourage participants to think about balance and harmony as they plan to add color and patterns to their containers. Repeating a shape or a color can add unity to the entire composition.

AFTER

While the containers are drying, ask the group to share the positive messages they wrote about their friends. This can be a very meaningful experience for all involved, promoting self-esteem and a sense of community within the group. Encourage participants to think of one positive affirmation about themselves to add to the messages their friends wrote. Discuss other ways group members can support and affirm each other.

Fruits of the Harvest: Painting a Still Life

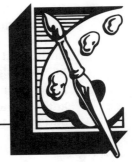

October

GOALS

- To gain awareness of the still life as an art form
- To paint a still life of seasonal fruits and vegetables
- To gain experience in gathering and setting up a still life suitable for painting

MATERIALS

- Images of still life paintings
- A variety of colorful fruits and vegetables of the season
- 12" x 18" white drawing paper
- Pencils
- Watercolors
- Brushes
- Containers for water
- See alternate supply list in adaptation box at the end of the activity

BEFORE

1. Set up a still life of fruits and vegetables before class begins. Interested participants may arrive early to assist with the set-up. It is okay to include other seasonal objects, such as an interesting Halloween mask or a cornu-

copia. A patterned tablecloth or sheet and a variety of containers may make the still life more dynamic.

2. Display visuals of paintings of still lifes to show the participants. Have participants examine the artwork, carefully pointing out exactly what they see. Ask questions such as:

   - What objects are in the still life?

   - What colors, lines, shapes, and textures are in the still life?

   - How did the artist arrange the composition?

   - How do shapes in the work extend out to the edge of the canvas?

   - How are objects in the still life portrayed realistically or how did the artist choose to represent them imaginatively?

3. After they have looked at several examples, have participants plan their own still life painting.

4. Select some of the fruits and vegetables from the still life and pass them around for closer viewing. Have participants describe the shapes and colors as carefully as possible. Stimulate a discussion on past experiences with objects from the still life. If there are gourds, what memories do people in the group associate with them? Pumpkins will undoubtedly trigger reminiscence about fall activities.

DURING

1. Hand out materials and encourage participants to think about what they want to include in their paintings. For example:

   - Will they include *all* of the objects or only a few?

   - Will they draw things to scale or will they exaggerate the sizes?

   - Will some objects overlap others? How will they handle this?

2. Ask participants to begin drawing on the white paper. Because many older adults with or without developmental disabilities are not confident about their drawing abilities, it is important for the instructor to walk around and interact with participants during this part of the lesson, offering encouragement and suggestions.

3. After outlining shapes and forms in the still life, participants are ready to begin painting. Watercolors are an excellent medium to use with a pencil drawing. Participants can add color without covering up the lines they have drawn. Encourage each person to think about what will be in the background of the painting. If they choose to leave part of the paper white, how does this work with the rest of the composition?

AFTER

After the still life paintings have dried, exhibit them at the facility. Simple mats made from construction paper can enhance artwork. Perhaps objects from the still life can become part of a table decoration at the facility during the coming week.

ADAPTATION

Encourage participants with limited vision to bring in objects from their rooms or their homes with which they are familiar. Have them select a few more objects from those displayed on the table. Encourage them to touch and, if possible, view closely all of the objects they will put into their picture. Instruct them to depart from the traditional pencil drawing followed by watercolor; instead, encourage them to experiment with collage materials (e.g., sandpaper, raised glue line, pipe cleaners, papers of very bright colors and rough textures) and to use Cray-pas and bright poster paints (fluorescent colors are appropriate here). Their works will be very different from those using only watercolors and will offer a good teaching opportunity for the rest of the participants to learn to appreciate differences among creations.

Mask Making (Part 1)

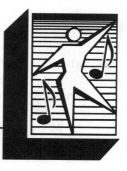

October

MATERIALS

- Construction paper
- Rubber bands
- Fabric scraps
- Glue
- Markers
- Feathers
- Scissors
- Paper plates
- Paint
- Glitter
- Yarn
- Any other mask-making materials

BEFORE

With the group, determine a theme for this unit on assuming a new persona with movement and masks. Have each person try out some movements that would go with the mask they will be making. Pass out supplies so that participants can make a mask of their choice. The mask can cover just the face or eyes or the whole body. Encourage the group to be creative. Suggest that they emphasize and exaggerate some of the characteristics they give to the costume so that the effect will be apparent.

DURING

Making masks can be an elaborate procedure or as simple as using aluminum foil that is first crinkled up and then pressed over the face to create the features. When painting on aluminum foil, add soap to the paint to make it stick. Three-dimensional forms such as balloons, basketballs, footballs, or paper plates can be used as the base for effective mask making using paper mache.

Tell participants to share their mask with others without telling them what they are supposed to be. Participants should try to guess what the other group members have become with their masks. Have participants think of movement to go with their new persona. Ask how their new characters might walk; have them experiment with different types of walking. Ask what sort of posture the characters might use and form a posture showcase in which characters, such as high-fashion models, walk a certain pattern while everyone else claps. Ask what sort of noises (or vocal styles) the character makes (or uses).

AFTER

Begin a group discussion by asking the participants to tell about their masks or costumes and how they got the idea for them. Ask the participants to respond in character to questions about their characters, such as:

- What do you do for a living?
- Where do you live?
- What are your friends, family, acquaintances, and affiliations like?
- What else should people know about your character's personality?

Suggest that the group try viewing the world during the coming week through the eyes of their new character. Ask them to think about and share during the next week what it was like to look at the world this way. What insights, revelations, and ideas did this activity reveal? Discuss any changes in their daily lives prompted by this experience.

ADAPTATION

Persons with dementia may need more direction in how to make a mask, what kind of character to give the mask, and how to dance as that character. Provide them with assistance in the mask fabrication process by ensuring that they have a buddy to help them, extra staff, or your own instruction. Suggest that they create a mask that exemplifies a state of being: happy, angry, sad, sleepy, shy, and so forth. Then the movement and dance in the mask will come more naturally.

Mask Making (Part 2)

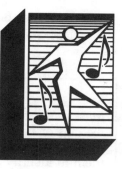

October

GOALS

- To give participants the chance to experience the leadership of a peer
- To develop concentration skills as participants are challenged to remember dance sequences
- To enhance self-esteem as participants perform for one another

MATERIALS

- Masks from previous lesson

BEFORE

Participants are encouraged to don their masks (made during the October dance lesson: "Mask Making [Part 1]") or exchange masks with others. Instruct everyone to find a partner.

DURING

1. Ask each pair to decide who will be the leader first and who will be the mover.
2. Tell the leader to make six movement commands to the mover that relate to the mask or costume.
3. Let the mover rehearse the pattern, then switch roles. Give each person time to rehearse the given movements.
4. Ask participants to perform their movements for the rest of the group. Encourage applause after every performance.

AFTER

Begin a group discussion by asking each of the participants questions about issues such as:

- How they felt when they moved with their masks on
- How they felt when performing in front of the group

ADAPTATION

Masks are an interesting topic for persons who have difficulty revealing their feelings or understanding who they are. Adapt this lesson by having the group make another series of masks—masks that represent themselves. Then direct them to identify at least four tendencies that they have. In the "During" section, ask participants to symbolize these tendencies in movement. The tendency to enjoy reading, for example, could be symbolized by a long reach up to a shelf (to get an imaginary book) and then a swift opening of the book. Ask participants to perform a dance with their masks in which they perform each movement eight times. Encourage the audience to clap after each performance. In the "After" section, discuss the value of "being oneself" when communicating with other people and, thus, dispensing of masks.

Healing Hands

October

MATERIALS

- Cassette player and cassettes

BEFORE

Have participants do the basic warm-up described in the Dance section of Chapter 3. Once completed, begin a discussion about pain and the constant aches one has as he or she grows older. Have everyone pick one main ache to concentrate on during the lesson.

DURING

With "aches and pains" always in mind, begin the following move to produce heat. Rub hands together for 8 counts and place hands on the location of the ache. Hold the hand on the ache for 8 counts. Do this 3 or 4 times. Pick eight of the participants' aches to warm. Combine a number of these different aches into a sequence. Repeat the sequence at least 2 times. Do not forget to rub hands together between each ache.

AFTER

1. Ask the group to divide into pairs. Ask one person to be the action and one person to be the mirror.

2. To accompanying music, slowly mirror the sequence of aches that were "danced" during the main activity.

3. Reverse roles with partners.

4. Ask participants to gather in a circle. Begin a group discussion by asking the participants such questions as:

   • How did it feel when you applied warmth to your ache?

   • Do the aches affect your life? How?

Encourage the group to continue to share their feelings about their aches and pains to someone they trust and to be sure to be a good "ear" and listen carefully and compassionately in return. Encourage them to increase their daily level of physical activity. They could participate in a daily activity with the person with whom they shared their feelings about their aches and pains. This could result in their having a sense of more control and of doing something about their aches and pains. Encourage the group to spend the necessary time giving proper care to their aches and pains.

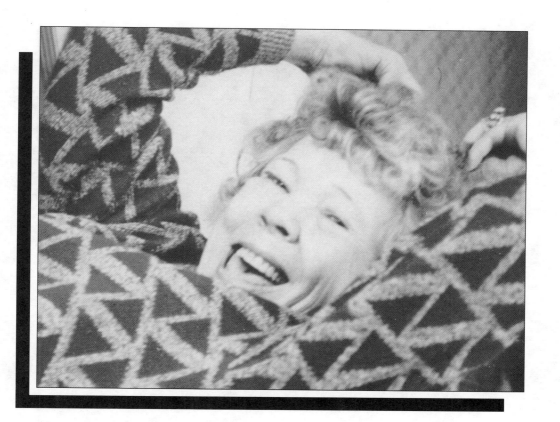

November

Themes:

Winter memories
Feasts and Thanksgiving
Gratefulness

Warm Up to Winter

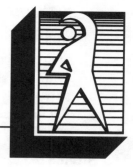

November

MATERIALS

- Cassette player and cassettes

BEFORE

Inform the group that November means cold weather. In cooler weather, it takes longer to warm up those stiff muscles and joints. Play music to accompany the following warm-up.

Warm-up

Seated

1. Tap the left foot 16 times, then the right foot 16 times.
2. Pick up the left knee and tap the left foot 16 times. Lift the right knee and tap the right foot 16 times.
3. Pat the left thigh with the left hand 16 times. Pat the right thigh with the right hand 16 times.
4. Try to pat the right thigh and tap the right foot at the same time. Try it with the left leg.

Standing

1. Stand and lift the feet high while marching in place.

2. Carefully swing the arms while marching.

3. Reach the arms out and clap while continuing to march in place.

4. Stand in place, bring arms out to the side, then lift them upward. As the song comes to an end, prepare to stretch.

Breathe

1. Step together to form a circle.

2. With feet shoulder-width apart and knees "soft" (slightly bent), roll the pelvis under and relax the arms by the sides.

3. Lift the arms up as high overhead as possible and inhale deeply. Return the arms to the sides and exhale. Repeat 4 times.

Stretch

Standing

1. Stretch arms overhead and stretch the fingers by extending the fingers as wide apart as possible, and then as close together as possible. Repeat these finger exercises out to the sides and then close to the body.

2. Extend the arms out in front and bring the arms up and down. As the arms move up, flex the hands down, and as the arms move down, flex the hands up. Repeat 8 times.

3. With arms relaxed by the side of the body, stretch the neck to one side, to the other side, then down in front.

4. Maintaining good body position, turn the head to see the neighbor to the right, then turn to see the neighbor to the left.

5. While turning the head to one side, exercise the eye muscles by looking as far as possible to that side. Repeat on the other side.

6. Place hands on shoulders and stretch elbows back as far as possible. If that seems too simple, try placing the hands behind the head and stretching the elbows back as far as possible. Repeat 4 times.

Seated

1. Sit in a sturdy chair with both feet flat on the floor. To strengthen the abdominal muscles, tighten them; feel the muscles tighten by placing the hands on the abdomen. Hold this for 4 counts, then release. Repeat 8 times.

2. Place both hands under the right thigh and bring the right knee in close to the chest. Continue to stretch the back of the leg (hamstring) by extending the leg as far as possible. Lower the right leg, extend it out, keep the knee slightly bent, and rotate the ankle 8 times in both directions. Repeat with the left leg.

3. To stretch arms and legs and work on coordination, stand next to a chair for support and extend the left leg and left arm in front and circle the ankle and wrist simultaneously. Repeat on the right side.

4. To finish stretching the arms, give yourself a hug to loosen the shoulders.

DURING

Suggest the group begin by using the resistance exercises that they worked on during lessons earlier this year. Remind them to keep their hands loose (no clenched fists). Play music with a lively tune and moderate beat.

1. In a standing position (if possible), extend the arms out to the side with palms facing the ceiling. Bring the hands in to the shoulders, then extend them once more. Try to keep the arms at shoulder height. Repeat 8 times. Repeat this exercise, alternating one arm and then the other. Repeat 8 times.

2. Repeat step 1, but turn the palms to the front. Repeat 8 times. Repeat this exercise, alternating arms. Repeat 8 times.

3. Repeat step 1, but bring the arms down by the sides, with palms facing the front. Imagine the elbows being pinned to the sides. Repeat 8 times. Repeat this exercise alternating arms. Repeat 8 times.

4. Bring the hands up to the shoulders and press the elbows behind the back. Extend the arms back as far as possible. This exercises the triceps. Repeat 8 times.

5. Begin with elbows by sides and hands by shoulders. Extend one arm up as the other stays in place. Alternate lifting one arm up overhead and then the other. Repeat 8 times.

Encourage the group to demonstrate the different ways that people keep warm when out in the cold. The most important thing to remember is to stay warm, so keep the group moving. Tell them to shake out their arms, starting with the hands and working up to shoulder rolls.

To continue moving for warmth, tell the group to do exaggerated marches, rubbing the hands together and patting the thighs. These three steps can turn into dance movements very naturally. Pick a song with a good beat and march 8 times, slide the hands back and forth 8 times, and pat the thighs 8 times. This is the winter warm-up! Try to encourage participants to create other moves, but continue with variations of these three if they seem to like them.

AFTER

1. Form a circle to begin the cool-down.

2. Sway from one side to the other, carefully swinging the arms from side to side.

3. Step forward and backward, carefully swinging the arms front and back.

4. Drop the arms by the sides and roll the shoulders, first in one direction, then in the other direction.

5. Finish by doing small lunges, first to the sides and then forward. Perform the lunges very slowly.

6. For a final stretch, give yourself a big hug to stretch the shoulders.

Harvest Time

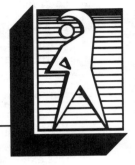

November

MATERIALS

- Cassette player and cassettes of peppy, spirited music

BEFORE

Inform the group that November means second harvest—time to get the last crops in before winter hits. Ask the group to think of the different activities used by farmers in their fields when harvest time arrives. Play music to accompany the following warm-up.

Warm-up

1. Imagine trying to walk through a field ready to be cut. Raise feet high while marching in place.
2. Extend the arms out in front while marching through the field.
3. Walk forward, continuing to move the arms out in front. Repeat this in reverse. Go slowly!
4. Stand in place and bring arms out to the side, then lift them upward. As the song comes to an end, slow to a stop and prepare to stretch.

Breathe

1. Step together to form a circle.
2. With feet shoulder-width apart and knees "soft" (slightly bent), roll the pelvis under and relax the arms by the sides.

3. Lift the arms up high overhead and inhale deeply. Return the arms to sides and exhale. Repeat 4 times.

Stretch

Standing

1. Stretch arms overhead and stretch the fingers by extending the fingers as wide apart as possible, and then as close together as possible. Repeat these finger exercises out to the sides and then close to the body. Repeat 8–10 times.

2. Extend the arms out in front, then bring the arms up and down. As the arms move up, flex the hands down, and as the arms move down, flex the hands up. Hold each stretch 10–15 seconds; repeat 8 times.

3. Stretch arms overhead and reach up higher with the right arm, then with the left arm. Hold each stretch 10–15 seconds; repeat 8 times.

4. With arms relaxed by the side of the body, stretch the neck to one side, the other, then down in front. Hold each stretch 10–15 seconds; repeat 8–10 times.

5. Maintaining good body position, turn the head to see the neighbor to the right, then turn to see the neighbor to the left. Hold each stretch 10–15 seconds; repeat 8–10 times.

6. Place hands on shoulders and stretch elbows back as far as possible. If that seems too simple, try placing the hands behind the head and stretching the elbows back as far as possible. Hold 10–15 seconds; repeat 8–10 times.

Seated

1. Sit in a sturdy chair with both feet flat on the floor. To strengthen the abdominal muscles, tighten them; feel the muscles tighten by placing the hands on the abdomen. Hold this for 4 counts, then release. Repeat 8 times.

2. Place both hands under the right thigh and bring the right knee in close to the chest. Continue to stretch the back of the leg (hamstring) by extending the leg as far as possible. Lower the right leg; extend it out, keep the knee slightly bent, and rotate the ankle 8 times in both directions. Repeat with the left leg.

3. To stretch arms and legs and work on coordination, stand next to a chair for support and extend the left leg and left arm in front and circle the ankle and wrist simultaneously. Repeat on the right side.

4. To finish stretching the arms, give yourself a hug to loosen the shoulders.

5. To loosen the back, slowly roll over, beginning with the head, until the hands touch the toes. Remember that this should be done while seated.

DURING

For the next 10–15 minutes, ask the group to demonstrate different movements used in harvesting. Some examples that come to mind are cutting wheat with a scythe, pitching hay with a pitchfork, loading bales onto a truck, and storing the hay in the barn. Urge participants to concentrate on moving, bending, and stretching during the entire period. Play music with a lively tune and moderate beat.

1. Cutting wheat: Swing the right hand down near the hip and step out on the left foot. Return to center. Repeat to the left.

2. Pitching hay: Put hands together and lunge forward on the left leg, swinging the hands down and up over the right shoulder. Repeat on the right leg.

3. Loading bales of hay: Bend the knees slightly and bring the arms in front close to the chest. Bring the arms up to shoulder height and punch out with both arms as if loading the bale on the truck.

4. Unloading bales of hay: Reach forward to grab a bale of hay. Bring arms back, close to the body at shoulder height, then turn to the right or left (alternate) and push arms out to drop the bale.

5. Try to come up with additional moves and continue moving until the end of the song.

AFTER

1. Form a circle to begin the cool-down.

2. Sway from one side to the other, carefully swinging the arms from side to side.

3. Step forward and backward, carefully swinging the arms front and back.

4. Drop the arms by the sides and roll the shoulders, first in one direction, then in the other direction.

5. Finish by doing small lunges, first to the sides and then forward. Perform the lunges very slowly.

6. For a final stretch, give yourself a big hug to stretch the shoulders.

Pilgrims

November

MATERIALS

- Cassette player and cassettes

BEFORE

Suggest that the group concentrate on imagining what life was like for the Pilgrims. Begin with a seated warm-up. Play music to accompany the warm-up.

Warm-up

Seated

1. Tap the left foot 16 times, then the right foot 16 times.
2. Pick up the left knee and tap the left foot 16 times. Lift the right knee and tap the right foot 16 times.
3. Pat the left thigh with the left hand 16 times. Pat the right thigh with the right hand 16 times.
4. Try to pat the right thigh and tap the right foot at the same time. Try it with the left leg.

Standing

1. Stand and lift the feet high while marching in place.

2. Carefully swing the arms while marching.

3. Reach the arms out and clap while continuing to march in place.

4. Stand in place, bring arms out to the side, then lift them upward. As the song comes to an end, prepare to stretch.

Breathe

1. Step together to form a circle.

2. With feet shoulder-width apart and knees "soft" (slightly bent), roll the pelvis under and relax the arms by the sides.

3. Lift the arms up as high overhead as possible and inhale deeply. Return the arms to the sides and exhale. Repeat 4 times

Stretch

Standing

1. Stretch arms overhead and stretch the fingers by extending the fingers as wide apart as possible, and then as close together as possible. Repeat these finger exercises out to the sides and then close to the body.

2. Extend the arms out in front and bring the arms up and down. As the arms move up, flex the hands down, and as the arms move down, flex the hands up. Repeat 8 times.

3. With arms relaxed by the side of the body, stretch the neck to one side, to the other side, then down in front.

4. Maintaining good body position, turn the head to see the neighbor to the right, then turn to see the neighbor to the left.

5. While turning the head to one side, exercise the eye muscles by looking as far as possible to that side. Repeat on the other side.

6. Place hands on shoulders and stretch elbows back as far as possible. If that seems too simple, try placing the hands behind the head and stretching the elbows back as far as possible. Repeat 4 times.

Seated

1. Sit in a sturdy chair with both feet flat on the floor. To strengthen the abdominal muscles, tighten them; feel the muscles tighten by placing the hands on the abdomen. Hold this for 4 counts, then release. Repeat 8 times.

2. Place both hands under the right thigh and bring the right knee in close to the chest. Continue to stretch the back of the leg (hamstring) by extending the leg as far as possible. Lower the right leg, extend it out, keep the knee slightly bent, and rotate the ankle 8 times in both directions. Repeat with the left leg.

3. To stretch arms and legs and work on coordination, stand next to a chair for support and extend the left leg and left arm in front and circle the ankle and wrist simultaneously. Repeat on the right side.

4. To finish stretching the arms, give yourself a hug to loosen the shoulders.

DURING

Play music with a lively tune and moderate beat.

1. March forward 8 steps; march backward 8 steps.
2. Throw a gun on the shoulder and repeat marches.
3. Aim and fire—you got a bird for the feast!
4. Grab the bird and swing it over one shoulder, then the other. Repeat each of these steps 8 times.
5. Repeat the above 4 steps together.

Other moves might include sweeping out the cabin, setting the table, basting the turkey, kneading the dough, or poking the fire. The most important thing is to enjoy the activity—tell the participants to have fun preparing for Thanksgiving.

AFTER

1. Form a circle to begin the cool-down.
2. Sway from one side to the other, carefully swinging the arms from side to side.
3. Step forward and backward, carefully swinging the arms front and back.
4. Drop the arms by the sides and roll the shoulders, first in one direction, then in the other direction.
5. Finish by doing small lunges, first to the sides and then forward. Perform the lunges very slowly.
6. For a final stretch, give yourself a big hug to stretch the shoulders.

ADAPTATION

Both the warm-up and stretching exercises may be done in a seated position. If lower extremities are mobile, marching may be done in place; if immobile, omit the marching and use the hands by bringing the hands up and down on the thighs or by alternately swinging the bent arms and pointing the fingers to the ears. The creative movements suggested for "During" may be done in a seated position.

Thankfulness

November

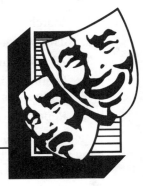

GOALS
• To increase nonverbal communications skills
• To encourage sharing
• To promote group interaction skills

MATERIALS

- Chalkboard and chalk or large piece of paper and marker

BEFORE

1. Discuss how November is a time to be thankful. Begin a group discussion by asking: What are some of the blessings you are thankful for? What are some of the things that you do not appreciate? Record answers in two columns on a large sheet of paper or on a chalkboard.

2. Lead the group in having each person pantomime something for which he or she is thankful and/or not thankful. The group will try to guess what each person is illustrating. Form the group into a circle so that everyone can see.

DURING

Divide the group into pairs. Instruct each pair to sit facing each other. One partner should tell a story about a time when he or she felt thankful or not thankful while the second person pantomimes the story. Once each person has finished his or her story, the pairs can switch roles. Allow adequate time for each person to pantomime.

AFTER

Discuss whether it is possible to be thankful for something, yet not be thankful for some aspects of it. Lead the group in discussing situations or objects that exemplify how things are made up of both the desirable and the undesirable.

Survival Skills

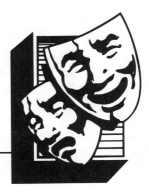

November

GOALS

- To increase communication skills
- To encourage mental flexibility
- To promote group interaction skills

BEFORE

Discuss the history of Thanksgiving. Encourage the participants to talk about how the Native Americans helped the Pilgrims and what survival skills they taught the Pilgrims. Ask the participants to describe a survival skill someone taught them.

DURING

Pairs of participants can dramatize how the Native Americans taught the Pilgrims to fish in streams using baskets and to plant corn using a dead fish put into each mound. Other teams of participants can show methods of preserving meat and fish by smoking. Others can explain how fruits can be sundried for preservation. Some participants can explain how to stalk deer and trap small game. Still other participants can enact teaching how to weave or how to chew deerskin soft for use in clothing.

In each team, one person should act out the role of the Pilgrim asking questions in order to learn, and the other person should act out the role of the Native American doing the teaching. Alternatively, participants could act out the survival skills someone taught them. Skits can be realistic or humorous.

AFTER

One topic for follow-up discussion is if and how some of these trapping and food preservation methods are still used today. Inquire if the participants have used any of them at any time in their lives.

Follow-up discussion might also focus on survival skills today. Discuss with the participants what survival skills they use in their lives. The discussion might come up with topics such as skills that protect us from outside harm, for example, locking doors and checking on elderly neighbors. Other survival skills are personal, such as avoiding or not overeating certain foods. Participants could share with each other what kinds of foods or drinks should be avoided.

Discussion might also focus on participants' favorite ways of preparing holiday foods. Inquire if there are differences in their recipes for pumpkin pie and cranberry sauce; how they know when the turkey is done; what they do with the leftovers, such as making turkey à la king using cream of mushroom soup or cooking the turkey to make a soup.

Preparing for Cold Weather

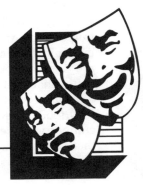

November

GOALS

- To stimulate cognitive functioning
- To increase group interaction skills
- To increase decision-making skills

MATERIALS

- Chalkboard and chalk or large piece of paper and marker

BEFORE

Discuss what people do to get ready for cold weather. Using a chalkboard or a large piece of paper, make a list of what the participants suggest. Some changes made during cold weather are activities are moved indoors, the garden is covered, and weather stripping is added to doors and windows. Ask participants to name activities that they still do or activities that they used to do several years ago.

DURING

Role-play how to get a home ready for winter with the help of a friend. In the skit, for example, pretend to climb ladders to clean out the gutters. One team could re-create things done in the kitchen. Another might enact things done in the garden. Use the list above to divide the group into teams for acting.

AFTER

After the skits, discuss how well the teams showed the different aspects of winter preparation. Ask if others use or used these methods or variations in their winter preparations. Discuss what things the participants could really do in the next few days to prepare their homes or rooms for winter.

Winter Birds: Creating Clay Tiles

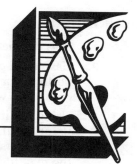

November

GOALS

- To create clay tiles
- To become more aware of winter birds
- To focus on birds as a theme in art

MATERIALS

- Visuals of birds and bird feeders
- One pound of clay per person
- Burlap squares or newspaper
- Toothpicks
- Drinking straws
- Plastic knives and forks
- Illustrations of decorative tiles
- Book of John J. Audobon prints (optional) or other illustrations of birds
- Bird feathers (optional)

BEFORE

1. Winter months offer a wonderful opportunity for bird watching. Stimulate a discussion about winter birds.
   - Do participants have bird feeders?
   - What kinds of birds to they see?
   - Do they have a favorite type and why?
   - What sort of seed attracts the most birds?
2. Show participants photographs of birds. If possible, show them examples of John J. Audubon prints. Encourage close observation of many kinds of

birds, noticing the variety of shapes, colorations, attitudes, and so forth. It would be excellent motivation if feathers were available to pass around for participants to touch and look at closely.

DURING

1. Pass out materials for creating tile reliefs of birds.

2. Have each person roll out a flat slab of clay and cut the outside edge of the desired shape with a plastic knife. This flat surface will provide the background on which each person will attach a bird form.

3. Using additional clay, have participants create a bird to attach to the tile. Point out the many successful approaches to solving this artistic problem. Participants may roll up a rounded form for the body of the bird, attach it to the clay tile, and then add the head, wings, tail, feathers, and so on. They may wish to put extra clay on the flat tile surface and then shape it into a bird with their fingers. Someone may prefer working with flat shapes, creating a bird that does not project off of the surface of the tile. Others may wish to draw directly into the tile with a toothpick. This project offers individuals the opportunity for self-discovery. What method do they prefer? What works best for them?

4. If participants wish to hang their tile reliefs on the wall, they will need to make two nail holes. Tell these participants to use a drinking straw and make openings in the top, being careful not to get too close to the edge.

AFTER

Store completed tiles in a safe place for drying. In 7–10 days they will be ready to fire.

Ask participants if they would like to plan a feeding station for birds at the facility. Is there a window that would offer a good view for potential bird watchers? Does anyone have binoculars that could be shared? Discuss who will coordinate buying birdseed and the feeder itself. What are some other ways to feed birds (balls of suet, pine cones spread with peanut butter)? Ask participants if they would like to keep a notebook handy to log the kinds of birds observed during the coming weeks.

Creating Placemats

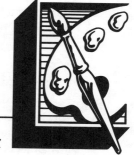

November

GOALS:

- To become familiar with feasts as a theme in art
- To reminisce about feasts and past Thanksgivings
- To create placemats for a Thanksgiving table

MATERIALS

- Images of feasts (Grandma Moses is a painter who often depicts large family gatherings. Norman Rockwell portrays family dinners and holiday feasts in his artwork. Examples of the work of these artists may be found at the local library.)
- 18" × 24" heavy white drawing paper
- Objects for printing (corks, erasers, vegetables, shells, cardboard, etc.)
- Sponges
- Tempera paints
- Styrofoam meat trays
- Rulers
- Pencils

BEFORE

Discuss what is meant by a feast. Focus on Thanksgiving feasts in particular and encourage reminiscence about past Thanksgivings.

Have visuals of feasts to share with participants. Carefully observe what is going on in the paintings, paying close attention to the types of food and table decorations, as well as interactions between the people involved.

What kind of Thanksgiving celebration will be held at the facility this year? What kind of special foods will be prepared? What sort of table decorations would create a festive atmosphere? Announce that this activity involves printing placemats that can be used at the facility or taken home for the holiday.

DURING

1. Place small sponges on Styrofoam trays and soak them in tempera paint. Prepare a variety of colors that are associated with fall, especially reds, yellows, and oranges.

2. Have participants look at several decorative placemats, paying attention to colors and patterning.
    *   What are the borders around the placemats like?
    *   Is there a large pattern or is patterning only in one area?
    *   How many colors were used?
    *   What is the dominant color?

3. Tell the group to begin creating their own placemats. If they wish to create borders, they may sketch them in with pencils. Have each person choose a few objects with which to print. Interesting patterns can be created using only one or two shapes. Vegetables cut in half, corrugated cardboard, corks, and flat shells are only a few suggestions of objects that make interesting shapes and patterns. Perhaps participants will want to bring things of their own to use for printing.

4. The instructor can demonstrate the stamp method of printing for the group. By gently pressing the object into the soaked sponge and then stamping it onto the paper, a clear image of the shape will result. Emphasize the importance of repetition to create patterns and variation to add interest.

AFTER

Let the printed mats dry. Additional color and detail will be added during the November art lesson: "The Environment: Completing Placemats." The completed mat can be laminated so that it will resist stain and can be wiped clean after use. Suggest that participants might want to make mats at home to give as gifts.

Have the group plan other table decorations for the Thanksgiving celebration at the facility. Does anyone have suggestions for music or entertainment that could add to the festivities? This could be a time for identifying special talents within the group. Encourage participants to contribute their unique skills to make this a meaningful Thanksgiving.

ADAPTATION

Individuals with severe mental challenge may stamp repeatedly in one area. To distribute the pattern over the entire placemat, it may be necessary for the leader or a friend to move the mat around in different directions so that stamping is move evenly distributed. These individuals may keep printing without realizing the necessity to re-ink the stamp between printings. Reminding the participant to re-ink after each stamping will result in clearer prints. An alternative method is to use a liquid shoe polish dispenser that fills itself upon being pressed. (See books in the Art Suggested Readings list at the back of this book by Anderson [1978], Clements and Clements [1984], Lindsay [1972], Ludins-Katz and Katz [1990], and Tilley [1975] for information on how to adapt materials for persons with severe impairments.)

Completing Placemats

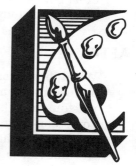

November

MATERIALS

- Samples of beautiful tableware (visuals from catalogs offer images of things that make a beautiful table setting)
- Printed placemats from November art lesson: "Creating Placemats"
- Watercolors
- Brushes
- Oil pastels
- Markers

BEFORE

Show the group examples of decorative china, napkins, and tableware. Discuss the importance of the environment and ask participants to make a list of things they do to make their surroundings more pleasant. What are some of the reasons people create an aesthetically pleasing table when they are preparing for a feast? Ask participants to share their experiences decorating tables.

DURING

Hand out materials and encourage participants to add details (and color if they wish) to the placemats they created during the November art lesson on placemats. If they created a patterned border, do they want to add color to the center of the work? Would their design be more effective if they outlined shapes in oil pastel or marker? If the design seems too plain, how will they go about adding other colors and shapes? This is a time for taking a second look and for making artistic decisions that will improve the work.

AFTER

When the placemats are complete, they may be laminated to protect them from stains and to allow for cleaning. A nearby school often has a laminating machine that they will be happy to let you use for a small fee. Once mats are complete, they can be displayed on the walls of the facility and then taken down for use during Thanksgiving.

Encourage participants to continue planning activities for their Thanksgiving feast at the facility. What are they doing during lessons from other disciplines (Drama, Dance, Fitness) about this holiday? Suggest visual art be included to make a big event out of Thanksgiving. Brainstorm for ideas.

Movement and Art

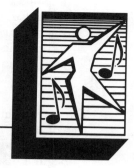

November

MATERIALS

- Art reproductions (from art books found in a local library)
- Original art (solicited from the participants)
- Long balloons
- One round helium balloon (large)
- Water-based markers that can write on balloons
- Props and artworks to be used to trigger expressive movement

BEFORE

Show participants the various examples of artworks and have them relate a story from their past or present to the artwork. If the art is an original made by one of the participants, ask about its history or reason for being made. Ask the participants to try to find patterns and other formal elements within the artwork.

DURING

1. Pass out the long balloons with markers and have participants make designs, patterns, and lines on the balloons that relate to the ones found in

the artwork. Have participants draw a symbol or pattern on the helium balloon.

2. With the balloons in hands, do simple movements. The balloons help participants move in a "larger" manner. The basic warm-up is okay here (see the dance section of Chapter 3). Use the design and artwork as resources to trigger movements, such as "uplifting," "strong," or "rapid"—whatever the participants see in the artwork and designs.

AFTER

Have participants tie the balloons to the larger helium balloon. This is now the "Tree of Life." The helium balloon should support the balloons while the other balloons should stop the helium balloon from drifting into the sky or ceiling.

Begin a discussion about the "Tree of Life." Where should it be displayed? What does it represent? Relate the "Tree of Life" back to the artwork used in the *Before* section of the lesson. Have the participants relate a personal experience to the "Tree of Life." Encourage them to notice and discuss the many patterns within the "Tree of Life." Encourage the participants to surround and move in a gentle manner around the "Tree of Life."

Movement and Mood

November

MATERIALS

- Chalkboard and chalk or large piece of paper and marker

BEFORE

Form a group of four to eight participants. Tell each participant to choose one of four words: "yes," "no," "why," or "because." Ask each participant also to choose one of three moods: sad, angry, or ecstatic. Solicit suggestions as to how one moves when feeling these emotions. Ask someone to write these suggestions on the chalkboard.

DURING

Tell one participant to begin to move and have the others gradually join in. Each participant should move in accordance with the mood chosen and may say the chosen word ("yes," "no," "why," or "because") whenever desired. The way the word is said should also reflect the chosen mood. The participants should play off each other's moods and words. Suggest that the participants change the moods, but not too often or arbitrarily. The word should never be changed. Stillness is allowed.

AFTER

Gather in a circle. Begin by asking each of the participants to think about and discuss:

- Why they selected their particular mood and word
- How it felt to have people respond to their mood
- What coping strategies they use when they feel sad

Suggest that throughout the week the group explore emotions by expressing and sharing moments when they feel sad, angry, or ecstatic with others. Ask them to watch how others show these feelings. Ask them to pay particular attention to the way their and others' emotions affect their movements and the language they use. Observations and insights by the participants about these topics, emotions, language, and movement should be focused on during the coming week.

Story from Movement

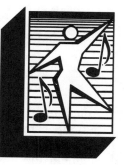

November

BEFORE

Invite the participants to form a large circle. Ask a volunteer from among the participants to shout out his or her name and then make a movement. Instruct the rest of the circle to shout out that same name and make the same movement.

DURING

1. Ask the participants to invent three movements. Teach these movements to everyone in the group.

2. After the first three movements are learned, add three more movements that the participants invent. Repeat the sequence several times. See how many different ways they can change the movement—slow, fast, loud, quiet. Let participants come up with their own ways of moving.

3. Go back to the original sequence and ask the participants to create a verbal phrase for each movement. The words may form a story.

4. Incorporate the words into the movement.

5. Select a volunteer participant. Ask the volunteer to shout a word at the group every other time you clap. The second time you clap, each member of the group instantly makes a movement to go with the word. It is important that the movement be one clear movement and not a lot of movements. Clap in a steady and slow manner.

6. Once everyone has the idea, change shouters, movers, and clappers.

AFTER

Begin a group discussion by asking how it felt to come up with a movement to a word that perhaps did not immediately bring a movement to mind. Did anyone make movements that had nothing to do with the word? What in life is similar to this situation? When are there times when we go ahead and act even if we do not understand the command? Discuss the merits of these actions.

ADAPTATION

Adaptations for persons with physical disabilities will generally follow one of two types: movement approximating that of others in the group (e.g., movement in a wheelchair or with the wheelchair) or the relegation of different tasks that augment the movement. Both of these approaches could occur in this lesson. When forming the movement sequence, create alternative, but similar, movements for those with physical disabilities. When the group is involved in the story creation part of the lesson, encourage those with physical disabilities to take the lead; perhaps a chorus could be created that narrates and introduces the action (similar to ancient Greek drama).

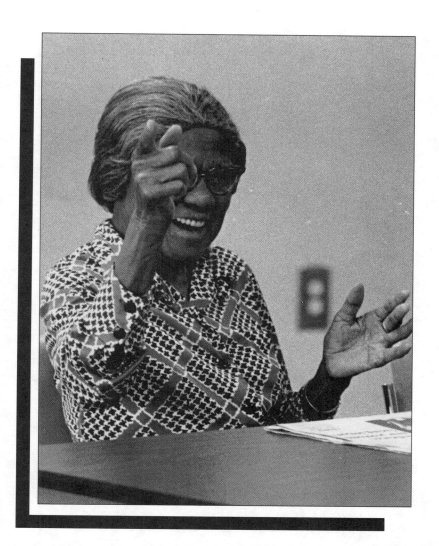

December

Themes:

Holidays and emotions of the season
Giving
Merriment
Joy and laughter

Decorating for Christmas

December

GOALS

GOALS

- To increase range of motion through activities simulating Christmas decorating
- To incorporate fitness activities with the Christmas traditions of decorating the house and the tree

MATERIALS

- Cassette player and cassettes

BEFORE

Remind the group that preparing for Christmas is always exciting. Perhaps one of the most enjoyable things is to decorate the house for this special holiday season. Suggest that there is nothing quite like the smell of a Christmas tree.

Warm-up

Inform the group that one needs to be in shape to do all that must be done to get ready for Christmas; therefore, participants must loosen and warm their muscles.

1. Walk around in a circle, carefully swinging arms back and forth. Hold the head high and stand tall. Walk around the room 2 times.
2. Turn and walk in the opposite direction. Walk the first circle on the toes. Use a normal step for the second circle.
3. Form a circle with all the participants and place hands on hips. Inhale and exhale slowly 2 times.
4. Raise arms outward from sides, then overhead while inhaling deeply. Exhale and lower arms to sides. Repeat 2 times.

Stretch

Neck: Suggest that participants pretend to look for just the right Christmas tree with each turn of the head.

1. Look left/look right: Turn the head and look over the left shoulder and hold 5 seconds, turn and look over the right shoulder and hold 5 seconds. Repeat 8–10 times.

2. Look down/look up: Look straight ahead, then lower chin to chest and hold 5 seconds. Repeat 8–10 times.

Shoulders: Notify participants that they now have the right tree. It is time to bring it home and decorate it.

1. Hand touches above head: Stand with hands together in front of thighs. Bring hands and arms as high above head as possible and return to starting position with a chopping motion (as if chopping down a tree). Repeat 8–10 times.

2. Arm reaches: Place hands on shoulders. Reach as far upward as possible, alternating arms and holding each stretch 15–20 seconds. Repeat 8–10 times.

Torso: Suggest that the group pretend to reach down for more ornaments.

1. Side stretches: standing next to a chair with feet shoulder-width apart and knees slightly bent, slowly lean from the waist toward the right and hold 15 seconds. After returning to an upright position, repeat to the left side. Alternate left and right 8–10 times.

2. Torso turns: Hold arms out from sides and slowly turn upper body to left and hold 15–20 seconds. Repeat turning to the right. Repeat 8–10 times.

Arms: Announce that the tree is ready for its star.

1. Triceps extensions: With the right arm bent and the right elbow pointed toward the ceiling, extend the right hand toward the ceiling until the arm is fully extended. Return to starting position. Repeat 5 times, then change to the left arm.

2. Arm presses: With both arms extended above the head, lower hands to shoulders and press back up above the head. Repeat 8–10 times.

Hips/Legs: Now ask the group to add finishing touches to the tree.

1. Half squats: Stand behind a chair for support, place feet shoulder-width apart, keep back straight, bend knees, and lower body halfway down. Return to standing position and repeat 8–10 times.

2. Toe raises: Stand behind a chair for support, slightly bend knees, then transfer weight to the balls of the feet. Hold for 15 seconds then return to starting position. Repeat 8–10 times.

3. Ankle circles: While seated, extend the right leg forward and begin turning the right ankle in circular motions. Change directions, then repeat with the left leg. Repeat 8–10 times.

DURING

Announce that the group will now make a wreath for the door. Play Christmas music and begin walking in a counterclockwise circle. As the participants make the wreath's circular form, lead them in the following exercises and repeat each one four times.

1. Circle both arms in front of the body, moving them in a clockwise direction.
2. Raise both arms in front of the body as high as possible, then return to starting position.
3. Clap both hands above head.
4. Clap both hands in front of the body.
5. Walk with weight on heels.
6. Walk on toes.
7. Alternate arms while reaching for the ceiling.
8. Push both arms out in front of the body, bring them in, then push them out again.
9. Bend knees and lower body every 4 steps.
10. Stop and face the center of the circle and tap the right foot 4 times, then tap the left foot 4 times.

Repeat all of the above movements or have participants move about to the music using any movements they choose. Try to sustain activity for a total of 15 minutes.

AFTER

Inform the group that one of the final things to do in decorating is to hang the mistletoe. After that, relaxation is in order.

1. Standing in place, alternately stretch arms overhead 4–6 times.
2. With feet shoulder-width apart, carefully swing arms forward and stand on tiptoes, then swing arms down and shift weight to whole foot. Repeat 4–6 times.
3. Walk slowly around the room (or in place).
4. Sit down in a chair and hold the left foot slightly off the floor. Circle the left foot in a clockwise direction, then in a counterclockwise direction. Repeat with the right foot.

Holiday Giving

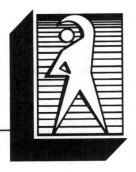

December

GOALS

- To foster the special feelings that come from giving
- To improve balance by walking within parallel lines
- To promote social interaction by engaging in contact activities

---

MATERIALS

- Cassette player and cassettes of Christmas songs
- Chalk
- Masking tape

BEFORE

Inform the group that one of the most meaningful aspects of the holidays is giving to others. Gifts may be toys, books, or articles of clothing, or they may be something simple and personal, such as a smile, a hug, or a helping hand. Ask participants to think of things that would make good holiday gifts.

Warm-up

Make parallel lines on the floor with chalk or put down strips of masking tape the length of the room that are approximately shoulder-width apart.

Invite participants to think of the feeling they get when they are choosing or making a gift for someone. Suggest that they imagine walking down a department store aisle looking for just the right gift.

1. Walk within the lines, carefully swinging the arms back and forth. Reverse position and walk back.

2. Continue walking in place and alternately extend arms straight out to the side of the body.

3. Standing in place, carefully swing both arms out, upward, then back down again.

Stretch

Neck: Offer the suggestion that a nice warm scarf makes a perfect gift.

1. Ear to shoulder: Tilt head so the left ear touches the left shoulder and hold 10 seconds; tilt head so the right ear touches the right shoulder and hold 10 seconds. Repeat 8–10 times.
2. Look down/look up: Lower chin to chest and hold 10 seconds, then raise chin so that head is back in line with the body. Repeat 8–10 times.

Shoulders: Inform the group that a favorite gift for children of various ages is a ball that can be tossed in the air, thrown, or caught.

1. Military presses: With both arms extended above the head, lower hands to shoulders and then press them back up above the head. Repeat 8–10 times.
2. Forward throws: With the right elbow bent and the right hand at shoulder height, extend the right hand and arm straight out as if throwing a ball. Repeat with the left arm. Repeat 8–10 times.

Arms: Suggest fishing rods as a gift. Remind participants what fun it is to throw out the line and reel in a fish.

1. Triceps extensions: With the right arm bent and the right elbow pointed toward the ceiling, extend the right hand toward the ceiling until the arm is fully extended. Return to starting position and repeat with the left arm. Repeat 8–10 times.
2. Arm curls: Extend arms down by sides with palms facing forward. Bring palms to shoulders, then return to starting position. Repeat 8–10 times.

Hands/Fingers: Inform the group that gloves not only warm the hands, but, when received as a gift, warm the heart, too.

1. Finger spreads: With elbows bent, and hands in front of the chest, spread fingers apart and hold 5 seconds. Bring them back together. Repeat 8–10 times.
2. Finger touches: Press the tips of each finger against the thumbs. Begin with the index fingers, then move to the middle fingers, ring fingers, and little fingers.

Hips/Legs: Inform the group that the dream of every child is to receive a gift such as a bicycle or roller skates.

1. Rocket kickers: With body positioned next to a chair for support, slightly bend knees and raise outside knee to hip level. Kick leg forward until fully extended, then bring back to bent knee position and return foot to floor. Repeat with other leg. Repeat 8–10 times.
2. 1-2-3 holds: Position body next to a chair for support. Carefully swing the right leg forward, then back, then forward again. On every third swing, hold the position 5–10 seconds. Switch legs. Repeat 8–10 times with each leg.

3. Crossovers: Stand behind a chair for support and slightly bend knees. Carefully swing the extended right leg across the body toward the left, then return to starting position. Repeat with the left leg. Repeat 8–10 times.

4. Bicycles: Sit in a chair. Extend the right leg forward, then bring it in to the chest. Extend it back out and lower it. Repeat with the left leg. Alternate legs for 8–10 repetitions.

Feet/Ankles: Mention that a pair of slippers makes one of the nicest gifts.

1. Ankle circles: While seated, rotate the right foot several times to the right, then to the left. Repeat with the left foot. Repeat 8–10 times.

2. Spread the toes: While seated in a chair, spread the toes of the right foot and then relax. Repeat with the left foot. Repeat 8–10 times.

DURING

Because the holidays are such a special time for children, ask the group to imagine how excited kids must be when they think about Santa; reindeer; sugar plum fairies; and gifts, such as toy trains, scooters, cycles, and toy soldiers. Play lively holiday music for the following exercises.

1. March in place, adding the following movements:
   a. Bend the right elbow and bring the right hand up to the shoulder. Lower it and repeat with the left arm. Alternate 8–10 times.
   b. Walk forward 4 steps and back 4 steps, then continue to walk in place.
   c. Bring the left arm straight out to the side from the shoulder, then bring it back to the shoulder. Repeat with the right arm. Alternate arms 8–10 times.

2. In single file, put the right hand on the shoulder of the person in front of you. Follow the "train" around the room.

3. In circle formation, perform the following movements:
   a. Step with the right foot sideways to the right, then slide the left foot to the right. Repeat to the left.
   b. Step left, kick the right leg to the left, step right, kick the left leg to the right.
   c. Walk in place 4 steps.
   d. Circle the right arm out to the right, and the left arm out to the left.
   e. Repeat the above movements 3 times.

Tell the group to think about gifts that cannot be bought, such as a visit, a greeting, or a hug.

AFTER

1. Line up in two lines facing each other about 6 feet apart. Walk toward the person directly opposite, then walk back to original place.

2. Swing the right arm slowly in front of the body up and down. Repeat 4 times, then change to the left arm and repeat 4 times.

3. Step forward on the right foot and swing both arms forward, then step forward on the left foot and swing both arms forward.

4. Stretch both arms out to the side, then cross them in front and reach around the back to give yourself a big hug.

ADAPTATION

Warm-up exercises may be adapted for those in wheelchairs by having them walk in place if mobility allows or by "walking" with the hands on the knees. For a more aerobic exercise, swing the bent arms.

All stretching exercises may be done in a seated position with the exception of the hip and leg exercises. Lower leg lifts and lower leg crossovers may be substituted if lower extremities are mobile; if not, these exercises may be done with hands and arms.

The *During* phase of the lesson may be altered by marching in place if mobile, or by marching with hands on knees or by alternately swinging the bent arms and pointing the fingers to the ears. When an exercise calls for forming lines and walking, include using the wheelchairs to form lines.

Thinking About Holiday Toys

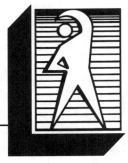

December

MATERIALS

- Cassette player and cassettes of Christmas songs

BEFORE

Tell the group that it is difficult to think of the winter holidays without thinking about children and toys. Of course, there are so many more types of toys now than in the past. Ask participants to imagine selecting a toy for a child.

Warm-up

Suggest that a good gift might be a music box with a ballerina, angel, or clown turning on top.

1. Touch steps: Lightly touch the ball of the right foot to the floor in front, then return the foot to center and touch the left foot in front. Carefully swing arms in a scissor movement in opposition to the foot pattern. Repeat sequence several times.

2. Flying: Extend arms at shoulder level. Move them up and down in a flying motion. Repeat 4–6 times.

3. Side bends: Bend the left knee, placing the lower left arm on the left thigh. Raise the right arm and bring it close to the right ear. Bend to the left and hold the stretch. Stand upright, bend the right knee, place the lower right arm on the right thigh, raise the left arm to the left ear, and bend to the right.

4. Walk in single file around the room, breathing in and out slowly.

Stretch

Neck: Suggest that another gift might be a baby doll whose eyes open and close and whose head turns in all direction.

1. Look up/look down: Lower chin to chest, hold for 10–15 seconds, then raise head so it is aligned with body. Repeat 10–12 times.
2. Ear to shoulder: Tilt head to the left (left ear to left shoulder) and hold 10–15 seconds; tilt head to the right (right ear to right shoulder) and hold 10–15 seconds. Repeat 10–12 times.

Shoulders/Arms: Suggest that someone might give a child a puppet that is controlled by strings.

1. Shoulder shrugs: Raise both shoulders toward ears, hold for 10–15 seconds, then return to starting position. Repeat 10–12 times.
2. Exaggerated shoulder rolls: With elbows bent, bring shoulders and elbows forward, then straighten arms and bring arms out to the side at shoulder height. Keep knees slightly bent. Repeat 10–12 times.
3. Double arm swings and reaches: Shift weight from one foot to the other in a rocking motion while swinging both arms high at right, then down and across body to shoulder height at left. Repeat 10–12 times.
4. Place hands on hips, then raise the lower arms out to sides until arms are straightened. Return to starting position. Repeat 10–12 times.

Torso: Mention that a rag doll is a toy to make or buy.

1. Straight back forward bends: Put hands behind lower back. Bend forward (keeping chin up, back flat, and knees "soft") and hold 10–15 seconds. Slowly straighten up to starting position. Repeat 10–12 times.
2. Side bends with arm lifts: Bend to the right side from the waist and slide the right hand down the right thigh while raising the left arm over the head. Return to starting position. Switch sides. Repeat 10–12 times.

Legs/Lower back: Inform the group that toy soldiers and skateboards are favorite Christmas toys.

1. March in place: Walk bringing knees up in front of the body. Keep the back straight and head held high while swinging arms back and forth.
2. Knee to chest: Sit in a chair, with feet flat on the floor. Bring one knee up, pulling it close to the chest with both hands positioned under the thigh. Return the foot to the floor and switch legs. Repeat 10–12 times.
3. Knee to opposite elbow: Sit in a chair with hands on shoulders. Bring the right knee up and turn the upper body to the right to touch the left elbow to the right knee. Return the right foot to the floor and switch legs.
4. Toe raises: Stand behind a chair with weight equally distributed on both feet. Shift weight forward to balls of feet, raising body upward. Return to starting position. Repeat 8–10 times.

5. Stork stands: Stand next to a chair for support. Raise the right foot slightly off the floor. Hold the position, then switch legs. Repeat 10–12 times.

DURING

Playing music such as "March of the Toys" from "Babes in Toyland," or other lively holiday music, organize the group into pairs. During the first musical selection, ask one person in each pair to perform active movements that the other person should try to mirror. During the next musical selection, have the other person lead. Movements can include:

1. Marching
2. Step together, step slide
3. Walking 4 steps forward then 4 steps backward
4. Arm swings
5. Shoulder rolls

AFTER

As the group performs the following cool-down exercises, ask them to think about the contented, relaxed feeling they have observed in children after they have played at length with new toys.

1. Take slow and deliberate marching steps in place.
2. Slowly swing arms forward, out, and down by sides.
3. Assume a forward stride position with right leg forward and hold. Repeat with left leg forward.
4. Slowly perform shoulder rolls in backward direction.
5. Extend arms overhead, stretch the body, then lower the arms and relax.

$\mathcal{E}$xpressing $\mathcal{A}$ppreciation

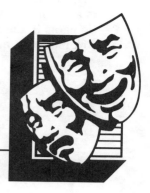

$\mathcal{D}$ecember

MATERIALS

- Items such as neckties, perfume, handkerchiefs, photographs from a vacation, ceramics
- Chalkboard and chalk or large piece of paper and marker

BEFORE

Discuss the importance not just of giving, but also of gracefully receiving. Discuss some of the silly, unwanted, unnecessary gifts that participants have received and for which they had to express thanks. Make a list of these gifts on the chalkboard or on a large piece of paper. Discuss their characteristics, their use, the personality of the giver, and how the gift fits into the holiday spirit. Discuss strategies for expressing appreciation to the giver. List these strategies.

DURING

As the leader, select one of the "gifts" and role-play thanking one of the participants for giving it. Then ask each participant to pick one of the gifts and role-play being given the gift. Following each skit, the actor should describe how he or she tried to express thanks, and the leader and the group should point out strategies that were used.

AFTER

Discuss the strategies for thanking givers that the participants used. See if there is any consensus on which methods of thanking are most successful. Urge participants in the days ahead to try out some new way of expressing appreciation. Ask if anyone has had a chance to express appreciation recently.

Capturing the Holiday Spirit

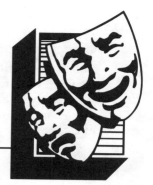

December

GOALS

- To recall humorous events
- To increase group interaction skills
- To increase social-planning skills
- To increase communication skills

MATERIALS

- Chalkboard and chalk or large piece of paper and marker

BEFORE

Using a chalkboard or a large piece of paper, make a list of activities done during the holidays: baking cookies, buying presents, shoveling snow, writing greeting cards, or receiving presents. Also list what participants enjoy and dislike about the holidays.

DURING

Divide the group into small groups to act out each of the scenes listed and the funny things that happen during each scene. For example, snow starting again just after the sidewalk has been shoveled clean, cookies burning in the oven, losing the holiday card list, or forgetting to send a greeting card to someone. Have each group brainstorm about what to include in the skit and who will play each role. Let them practice their skits.

Suggest that each group may want to act out a story; create a small puppet show; pantomime a holiday song or events such as decorating the tree, lighting the menorah, breaking a piñata, opening presents, and so forth. Help each group to include movement and action in their performance. Ask each group to select a member to serve as the narrator for the group.

AFTER

Following the skits, discuss each actor's performance and the interactions among the participants. Discuss how each participant's personality came out. To focus on the present and to extend the activity outward, encourage the participants to think about what will happen in the next few days. Encourage them to make connections between what was seen in the skits and what happens in real life.

Acting Out Christmas Carols

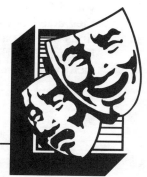

December

GOALS

- To increase group interaction skills
- To increase social-planning skills
- To promote socialization and peer interaction

MATERIALS

- Cassette player and cassettes of Christmas carols
- Video camera (optional)
- Simple props (Christmas theme) (optional)
- Television (optional)

BEFORE

Discuss how Christmas carols can be acted out. Determine if certain carols have more dramatic potential than others (e.g., "The Night Before Christmas" versus "Rudolph the Red-Nosed Reindeer"). Accompany the brainstorming about how to act out the carols by playing carols. Stop the music when necessary to point out some action, for example, "a pipe held tight in his teeth," and ask the participants how they could act this out.

DURING

Participants for each carol can lip-synch to the recording or sing along. As a way of providing participants with feedback on their performance, a video camera can be used to record an in-process rehearsal as well as the final performance. Alternatively, the entire group can sing along as one person or a small group performs the carol.

AFTER

Discuss the performance of each carol. If a video has been made, the group can watch the video of the performance and give participants praise on how well they acted out certain gestures. Ask if carols are sung at participants' celebrations and if participants have a chance to sing along. If the participants are interested, perhaps the group could give a "concert" on another wing of the facility or go from room to room singing carols.

Gift Giving: Printmaking (Part 1)

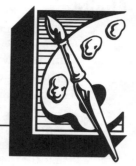

December

GOALS

- To focus on and reminisce about the concept of "holiday giving"
- To experience printmaking by creating cards, invitations, or program covers for the December drama activity, "Capturing the Holiday Spirit"

MATERIALS

- Examples of greeting cards
- Rectangles of Styrofoam (These can be cut from meat trays to the size of 3½" × 6" or 4" × 9" in order to fit standard envelopes.)
- Pencils
- Newsprint cut to size 3½" × 6" or 4" × 9"
- Standard-size envelopes

BEFORE

Discuss memories of holidays, such as Christmas and Hanukkah. Encourage "giving to each other" by the act of sharing these memories. Stimulating topics might be past holiday experiences, such as the group's earliest Christmas or Hanukkah, or the most extravagant or memorable gift they ever received or gave.

One of the most important aspects of the holiday season is gift giving and remembering friends and family. Each participant should choose an item he or she wants to make as a gift for someone. Making invitations to the show "Capturing the Holiday Spirit" (see page 385) for their "significant others" and/or sending greeting cards are great ways to let other people know you are thinking about them.

Show the group examples of attractive holiday greeting cards and have the group look closely at how they were designed. Is there a narrative image on the front of the card? Are holiday symbols used as a design motif? Ask the participants if the colors work well and why.

DURING

1. Pass out materials for preparing a printing plate. The printing plate should be about ¼" smaller on all sides than a standard envelope and the newsprint on which designs are to be sketched should be the same size as the printing plate.

2. Provide newsprint for sketching design ideas for the front of a holiday card.

3. Once they have worked out exactly what they want to print, the participants are ready to draw the image directly onto the Styrofoam plate with a pencil. Press hard enough to leave a strong mark indented, but not so hard that the pencil goes through the Styrofoam. The line should be impressed deeply enough to feel "bumpy" to the tips of the fingers. Remember that the image drawn onto the plate will print its opposite. Letters must be written backward in order to be read when printed. In other words, the printing plate is a mirror image of the final printed card. Thus, the letters must be formed on the Styrofoam mirror-backward.

AFTER

Put completed plates in a safe place for the actual printing during Part 2 of this lesson. If the participants intend to send the cards, encourage them to think about and make a list of names and addresses of people whom they will greet with their cards. If the prints will be invitations or covers, discuss the project that the art will announce.

ADAPTATION

Persons with developmental disabilities or dementia may need help in forming the address list of the recipients. A family member may be able to provide this information.

Gift Giving: Printmaking (Part 2)

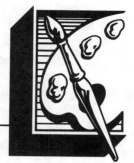

December

GOALS

- To print holiday cards, programs, or program covers
- To focus on the idea of giving to others

MATERIALS

- Colored construction paper
- Heavy white drawing paper
- Styrofoam printing plates made during the December art lesson "Gift Giving—Printmaking (Part 1)"
- Water-base printing ink
- Three or four brayers (rubber rollers used for printing, which can be purchased at any art supply store)
- Uncut Styrofoam meat trays
- Holiday cards
- Two long tables
- Newspapers

BEFORE

This lesson is a continuation of the December art lesson: "Gift Giving: Printmaking (Part 1)," in which participants designed printing plates for holiday cards. It would be helpful to present a variety of holiday cards and focus on the choice of colors and why they do or do not work well. Tell the group that they will be choosing their own colors for their designs.

Cover two long tables with newspapers for this lesson. One table is needed to place wet prints to dry and the other will be used for printing.

DURING

Ask participants to choose several pieces of colored construction paper and white drawing paper on which to print. Tell them to fold the paper in half. It is important for participants to have everything they need before beginning to print.

1.   Squeeze printing ink on one long thick line at the top of the Styrofoam tray. Demonstrate how to ink the brayer by putting it in the ink and then rolling and pulling the ink down onto the tray. The entire brayer should be coated evenly with ink.

2.   Roll the brayer across the printing plate, covering all parts with ink.

3.   Place the inked plate face down on the front of the card and gently rub the back with the fingers, being careful not to wiggle the plate and smudge the design.

4.   Pull the paper off and place the wet card on the table to dry.

5.   Re-ink the brayer and continue printing until all cards have been made.

AFTER

Let prints dry and then distribute them to participants. What message would they like to put inside their cards? Perhaps they would like to share ideas or write jingles that would be appropriate for the holiday season. If someone has difficulty writing, ask another participant to assist. Encourage participants to talk about the people to whom they are sending their cards.

ADAPTATION

Due to the messy nature of printing ink, extra staff or responsible group members may need to be available to help participants with developmental disabilities or dementia.

The Nutcracker: Painting to Music

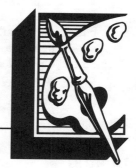

December

> ## GOALS
>
> - To promote awareness of the importance of play
> - To enjoy Tchaikovsky's ballet "The Nutcracker"
> - To reminisce about favorite toys
> - To paint to music

MATERIALS

- Cassette recorder
- A cassette or video of Tchaikovsky's ballet "The Nutcracker"
- An illustrated version of "The Nutcracker" (e.g., *Nutcracker* [1984] by E.T. Hoffman [New York: Crown])
- Books with illustrations of paintings by Van Gogh to use as examples of color representing strong emotions
- Books with illustrations of paintings by contemporary artists such as Robert Motherwell and Jackson Pollock, who use lines as important elements to express movement and emotion
- Long white butcher paper
- Block tempera paints
- Brushes
- Water

BEFORE

Research shows that play is important to the well-being of both children and adults. A playful attitude fosters creativity, allowing individuals to approach problems and tasks with a sense of freedom and flexibility as they look for solutions and new ways of doing things. The holiday season provides an opportunity for talking about the importance of play and having fun.

Tchaikovsky's ballet "The Nutcracker" is based on the story of a child's favorite toy. Share illustrated books of the story with participants. A video of the ballet itself could be shown at the facility during the week. Initiate a dialogue about memories of favorite games and toys. What sort of games did participants enjoy playing as children? Do children still play these games today? Ask participants how things are different today. Do group members have grandchildren and, if so, what kinds of things do they play with?

Announce that this art lesson focuses on "having fun." Participants will paint in response to music from "The Nutcracker."

DURING

Cover a long table with white butcher paper, or, if space allows, have white paper taped along a wall. Participants need as much room as possible to allow for a full range of motion.

Show illustrations of several paintings that evoke a mood. These can be abstract designs or realistic images. Using these images, discuss the power of color to affect feeling. Do participants associate certain colors with feelings? Think of common expressions that relate to this phenomenon: "Feeling blue," "Red with anger," "Green with envy," "Having a blue day." Discuss the ability of lines to express movement. Ask the older adults what kind of movement wavy, curved, straight, or jagged lines express.

Play music from Tchaikovsky's "The Nutcracker." Select a variety of moods and tempos and ask participants to close their eyes and concentrate on the music. What feelings does it evoke? Is it sad? Is it lively? As the group listens to the music, tell them to paint their own feelings and responses to the music using block tempera paints. Encourage large motions (moving the entire body if necessary) that reflect the tempo of the music and use of color to reflect the mood. Sometimes it is helpful to close one's eyes in order to heighten receptivity. The main purpose of this lesson is to have fun, relax, and "lean into" the sound.

AFTER

Have the group step back and look at the mural they have created. Can they see areas that reflect a similar response to the music? Do some of the colors and lines seem to reflect an upbeat mood and tempo? What is the overall feeling created by the mural? Inquire if the participants had fun during the process of musical response painting.

Suggest that group members bring any nutcrackers or toys they may have collected to the center for display during the holiday season.

Something About Us in Movement

December

GOAL

- To provide an opportunity to make a dance sequence from personal movement styles

---

BEFORE

Have groups of about eight participants sit in a circle and do a basic warm-up as described in the Dance section of Chapter 3.

DURING

1. Help participants to come up with a movement that describes their personality, hobbies, or values. It could be a hug, punch, smile, carpentry movement, cleaning movement, and so forth.

2. Have the group put the eight movements together. The eight movements should correspond to 8 counts. Count out the dance and have the group perform it. Repeat.

3. See how the dancers change the movement when it is counted differently. Advise the group to make the movement larger or smaller, happier or sadder, choppier or smoother.

4. If time allows, choose another group of eight people and create a second dance.

AFTER

Gather in a circle. Begin a group discussion by asking each of the participants:

- How does the movement you selected correspond with your personality?
- Was there a common theme to the movements?
- Do we all make the same movement the same way?

- Does the movement selected suggest something to us about how we might do something differently?

Suggest that throughout the week the group watch the movements of the many different people involved in their daily lives. Suggest they they select a certain activity that they see many people do (e.g., walking, eating, opening doors) and watch for individual variation. The next time the group meets, ask participants to share their findings. How do people of different personalities do the same activity?

Leading Involuntary Body Movements

December

MATERIALS

- Chalkboard and chalk or large sheet of paper and marker

BEFORE

Ask the group what movements people make that are involuntary. Make a list of these movements on the chalkboard or a large sheet of paper. Change these involuntary movements into commands. The list may look like:

- Laugh
- Giggle
- Sob
- Shiver
- Whimper
- Cough

- Sneeze
- Shake
- Choke
- Tickle
- Itch
- Yawn

DURING

1. Select a leader. The leader represents the need to cough, laugh, giggle, and so forth. Direct the leader to call out an action from the list above.

2. Instruct the participants to begin by "(involuntarily) performing" the action as literally as possible. Suggest that they begin to abstract it by using as many parts of the body as they can, clarifying the rhythmic pattern or exaggerating the movement. Participants may suggest other actions.

3. After the leader has given all the commands at least once, choose a new leader. Everyone should get a chance to be the leader.

AFTER

Ask the group if by performing any of these movements they really felt the accompanying emotion. For example, when they yawned, did they feel sleepy? Inquire if they think that it is odd that they can perform these actions with complete realism when the body needs to, but it is very difficult to make the movement seem real when the body does not need to perform it. In other words, everyone knows how to laugh when one thinks something is funny, but it is hard to laugh when one is not amused. Suggest that throughout the week the group look for times when they or others perform involuntary actions. Also, encourage participants to take a close look at people when they make these kinds of movements. Often, the "command" completely overcomes the body and stops all other functioning. Many people have very odd ways of yawning, laughing, and itching. Some people sneeze two or three times in a row while others only sneeze once.

A Dance in Santa's Spirit

December

GOAL

- To become aware of the many emotions of the Christmas season

MATERIALS

- Cassette player and cassettes of cheery holiday songs

BEFORE

Have the group sit in a circle and discuss the character of Santa Claus. Did they believe in Santa when they were kids? How has the myth of Santa changed over the years? Ask them to explain what Santa Claus is like as if they were telling someone who did not know.

DURING

As a group, pick four or eight movements that Santa Claus might make. Ask the group to put the Santa movements together into a dance. Perform the dance several times or have each member do a Santa dance for the rest of the group. Encourage clapping after each performance.

Suggest that the group think of different ways to be Santa Claus. Could Santa be very thin? Could Santa be a woman? How would Santa move if he or she got stuck in a chimney, if his or her sleigh were out of control, or if he or she bounced everywhere?

AFTER

Certainly a central characteristic of Santa is generosity—his job is to give gifts. Ask the participants what gifts they will be giving this holiday season. Have they purchased or made them already, or do they still have some work ahead of them? Who will be the recipients of the gifts? Will any of the recipients really think the gift came from Santa? If the group still has some shopping to do, perhaps this would be a good time to make plans to go on a group shopping spree. Perhaps there is a local parade in which the real Santa Claus will appear! Were there any other myths that you had to unlearn the hard way, such as "marry a prince on a white horse"?

Field Trip to a Local Art Museum

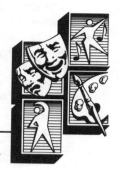

Appendix

A field trip to a local museum can be a very enriching activity for older adults with and without disabilities. It provides them with the opportunity to view works of art and it allows them to interact with their community. If possible, allow the older adults to mingle with other visitors and view the museum at their own pace. Major exhibitions often offer guided tours to aid viewers in the appreciation of the show. These are wonderful opportunities for older adults with and without disabilities to partake together in cultural events, bringing their unique gifts of wisdom and insight. Their participation adds a much needed dimension to a society that often isolates and devalues its older population. Museum field trips can bring older adults into the cultural mainstream, allowing them both to be enriched by and to enrich society through their participation.

Ideally, a museum field trip should consist of four major components:

- Planning phase
- Pre-museum lesson
- Museum visit
- Post-museum lesson

Each of these stages is designed to strengthen the experience as a whole, making it as meaningful as possible for the participants. If time is a problem, the last three components can be accomplished in 1 day, but it would be preferable to implement each one on a separate occasion, allowing participants to process the information and give them time to enjoy each experience fully.

THE PLANNING PHASE

The logistics of organizing the field trip may take several days and should begin 2–3 weeks before the actual visit. It will be necessary to contact the museum and talk with the staff member in charge of scheduling field trips. Some important points to cover are:

✔ *Set up a suitable date and time for the visit and determine how long it should last.*

✔ *Obtain information on the current exhibit.*   Check with the education staff to see what visuals the museum may have to help prepare the group for their museum visit. A catalog or slides of the art objects would be helpful to preview the work and to provide interesting background information. Perhaps a large poster of artwork from a current exhibition is on sale in the museum shop and could be displayed at the facility before and after the field trip.

✔ *Find out if there is an appropriate suitcase tour that could be used at the facility for the pre-museum lesson.*   The purpose of the suitcase tour is to present an interesting lesson and to allow participants to see actual objects or visuals that are brought to them in the suitcase. These tours can be brought to the facility by a museum volunteer called a docent. Even if the suitcase tour does not focus on the particular exhibit the group is going to see, it may provide them with general background knowledge that will enrich their museum experience. There are a variety of themes found in suitcase tours. Some of them include:

1.   Basic elements of design (color, line, shape, texture, form)

2.   The art of a particular culture (e.g., African art, Indian art)

3.   A movement in art (e.g., Impressionism, Cubism, Realism)

4.   Art as a way of expressing emotion

5.   A type of art (e.g., landscape, portraiture, still life)

A museum volunteer who is trained in the museum's collections would be very informative in preparing the group for their field trip. However, a facility staff member can do an excellent pre-museum lesson if the proper information and visuals are available. This person has the advantage of knowing his or her own particular group and how they learn best.

✔ *Let the museum know what special arrangements may need to be made for individuals with disabilities.*   Special arrangements that may need to be made include assistance with folding chairs. Questions to ask participants to determine their special needs include:

1.   Who will need help getting up steps?

2.   Will anyone need help riding in an elevator?

3.   Is everyone able to stand for 15 minutes at a time?

4.   Who will need a chair or a bench to sit on?

5.   How could the museum help you enjoy your visit?

Plans for getting the group in and out of the museum and for making them comfortable while they are there should be made well in advance of the field trip.

✔ *Ask if specially trained museum volunteers (staff members or docents) might be assigned to help take the group through an exhibition.*   Because one of the major functions of a museum is to provide an enriching educational experience for the public, museum staff members are usually friendly, cooperative, and eager to do what they can to work with groups with special needs.

PRE-MUSEUM LESSON

The pre-museum lesson is designed to prepare participants for their trip to the museum. Many older adults and adults with disabilities have never been to a museum. They will need a great deal of information to allay any fears they may have and to maximize the experience. Before beginning the lesson it is important to introduce yourself to the group, if they do not already know you. Tell them who you are and the purpose of the lesson. The more comfortable the participants are with you, the more at ease they will be on the day of the field trip.

The objectives of the pre-museum visit are:

1. To teach participants about the functions of a museum
2. To present pertinent information on the exhibit
3. To inform participants of the details of the field trip

Function of a Museum

Explain the purpose of a museum to the participants. It is a place that collects, takes care of, and exhibits objects that are historical, beautiful, and/or educational. There are many kinds of museums; they exhibit materials on such topics as science, natural history, and art. Some small local museums have works of art that belong to the museum and are stored there. They also may display visiting art shows.

Some questions to prompt dialogue about museums include:

Who has been to a museum?

Who has been to this museum?

What is your favorite kind of artwork (painting, sculpture, etc.)?

Where outside of the museum do you think you can find works of art?

Information on the Current Exhibit

The pre-museum lesson is the time to use whatever visuals or information are available from the museum about the exhibition. The more visuals available, the better prepared the group will be to enjoy the artwork. This also can be a time to heighten anticipation and get everyone excited about the field trip and what they will see!

Teaching Strategies

✔ *Keep it simple.*   Older adults with or without disabilities may not have a broad enough vocabulary to understand art terminology. Use language that is appropriate for them.

✔ *Ask questions to prompt dialogue.*   Never assume the group knows something. Often it is necessary to begin with the basics. If the field trip is to an exhibit of African art, use a map of Africa and start with a geography lesson. Explore questions such as: Where is Africa? How would you get there from here? How large is Africa compared to the United States? What part of Africa does this artwork come from?

If the field trip is to an exhibit of Impressionist paintings, begin with a simple lesson on color observation. Ask questions such as: What colors do you see in the sky? How do those colors change with the time of day? What are the colors in the morning? At midday? In the evening? How could you capture those colors in a painting? What colors can be made by mixing the three primary colors (red, yellow, blue) together?

✔ *Focus on a few major works in the exhibit.* There may be so many art objects that the viewers could become overwhelmed. It is better to concentrate on a limited number and then allow time for the group to look at others on their own.

✔ *Find ways to help participants connect with artwork though reminiscence, expression of emotion, and close observation of the elements of design.*

1. *Reminiscence:* Often artwork can trigger memories for older adults with or without disabilities. Allowing them to reminisce about important events in their lives is a valuable part of the life review process. The more personal connections they make, the more meaningful their experience will be. For example, if the group consists primarily of farmers or gardeners, find art objects that relate to agricultural activities. A sample of open-ended questions that provide the viewer with an opportunity to reminisce and make personal connections include: What is going on in this painting/sculpture/drawing? How does it remind you of something you have seen or done before? Where have you ever seen an animal such as this one? This is a scythe used by the Egyptians. How does it compare to the harvesting tools you have used?

2. *Expression of emotion:* Is the artwork expressive of emotion? If so, help the group to understand and empathize. Does the artwork elicit an emotional response in the viewer? Help the group to identify this response exactly. Making a connection with a work of art on an emotional level can make the encounter especially meaningful for the viewer. Some questions to encourage dialogue might include: How do you think the person in this sculpture is feeling? Why? When have you felt this way? Color can convey emotion. How did the artist use color in this painting to create a mood? How does it make you feel? Would you like to imagine what could happen next to the person in this artwork? You can change the feeling that the artist has portrayed if you wish.

3. *Elements of design:* Looking at art through the elements of design can also capture a group's interest. Line, shape, color, form, and texture provide a visual vocabulary that can prompt close observation and interesting discussion. Help the group become aware of these elements by asking such questions as: What is the main color in this painting? What is the brightest color? How many different shades of blue can you find? Where are the curved lines in this drawing? What other kinds of lines do you see? Let's make a list of every kind of line the artist has used. Look around and see if you can find any of these lines on or near you. What is the largest shape in this painting? How many circles can you find? Which shape has the artist used most often? Something that is three-dimensional has form. It has

height, width, and depth. (Have an example of an object to illustrate this idea.) Where in this painting do you see any objects that have forms? What do the forms in this sculpture look like? For example, are they rounded or do they have straight edges? If you could step into this painting and touch something, how would it feel? What words can you think of to describe the texture?

These questions will encourage close viewing and help your group to really *see* a work of art. Participants will make many discoveries on their own with a little encouragement.

Details of the Field Trip

Present logistical information about the actual field trip. Answer *when, who, what, how,* and *where* questions as simply as possible, making sure to include every detail of the trip. Here is an example of appropriate dialogue:

1. *When:* "We will be leaving from the facility Thursday morning at 10:00."

2. *Where:* "Gail will drive the van to the museum, which is located on Jackson Street."

3. *How:* "We will go in the back of the museum. (The staff will accompany those who would like to go up in an elevator.) Gail will park the van and the rest of the group will go in the lobby at the entrance."

4. *Who:* "Mrs. Harvey is a docent who does volunteer work at the museum and will meet us inside to help in any way she can. She knows a great deal about the artwork there."

5. *What:* "The Cameroon exhibit is in one large room to the right as you enter the front of the museum. Objects are out in the open, not under glass, and the museum has asked visitors not to touch anything to avoid damage. We will stay together as a group and look at eight of the artworks, then you will be able to walk around the room and look at whatever you want."

For many participants, a trip to a strange and unfamiliar place can be frightening unless they know exactly what to expect. Be prepared to answer any questions the group may have about the trip to increase their sense of comfort and well-being. Museum staff are usually very friendly and eager to help visitors feel at ease.

FIELD TRIP TO THE MUSEUM

If the pre-museum lesson has been informative, participants should be fully prepared for the actual field trip. It is a good idea to review the details of the trip, reminding the group of exactly where they are going, how they will get into the museum, and what they will be seeing.

The objectives of the field trip are:

1. To transport older adults with and without disabilities to and from the museum as safely and smoothly as possible

2. To make the group aware of appropriate museum behavior

3. To help participants encounter artwork in a meaningful way

At the Facility

After reviewing the logistics of getting to and from the museum, remind the group of proper museum behavior. If this is their first visit, they may be totally unfamiliar with certain rules and regulations. The following guidelines should be observed.

1. Works of art may be "touched" with eyes only. The museum is trying to preserve the objects on display; fingerprints leave dust and oil on the artwork.

2. The museum provides a nonsmoking environment for works of art. If some participants enjoy smoking, they should do so before or after the visit.

3. In order to protect art objects from damage, the museum asks that visitors keep sharp objects in their purses or pockets.

4. If a guide is taking the group through the exhibit, participants should respect the rights of others to listen and speak in a moderate tone of voice.

5. The group should stay together during the first part of the visit. This will enable participants to see the objects the group has studied during the premuseum lesson. Then they can look around on their own.

At the Museum

Take the group into the museum and directly to the particular exhibition that was chosen. Often older adults do not have the physical stamina to stay on their feet for long periods of time, and it is necessary to make the most of every moment. If the museum staff is prepared for the visit, they should be ready and waiting for the group to arrive.

Either the leader or a docent has familiarized herself with selected objects in the exhibition and is prepared to help the group interact with them. Here are some tips for making this part of the field trip successful:

1. Let the museum staff know who is responsible for the tour and what the goals, methods, and objectives are for the group. If a docent or staff member has been asked to be on hand, will he or she be most helpful as an assistant and facilitator or should he or she take charge?

2. Be sure that any chairs that are required are placed so that individuals with disabilities can see most of the artwork selected for viewing. If seating is available in the gallery, many participants may choose to sit rather than walk around and look at the entire exhibit.

3. Be flexible! Things will probably not go exactly as planned, so be prepared to "go with the flow" if necessary.

4. Promote game-like activities for closer observation of artwork and enjoyment of participants. Questions such as "How many faces can you find in this mask?" or "How many different shades of red can you discover in this painting?" are good ways to get participants to use all of their powers of observation.

5. Develop group management techniques that are age-appropriate. Some older adults, both with and without disabilities, will talk in spite of requests to the contrary.

6. Be gentle, go slowly, and be respectful of feelings. Going to a new and strange place can be unsettling for some individuals. The quality of the experience is far more important than the quantity of artwork encountered.

7. Allow time for the group to wander freely through the gallery and make their own viewing choices. After participants have seen the selected exhibition objects, they may want to go back and spend more time with certain pieces of art, or maybe venture off on their own to see something entirely different.

8. Distribute any available brochures about the exhibit to group members before leaving the museum. This is a good way for participants to have a visual reminder of the field trip that they can share with friends and family.

9. Allow time for a bathroom break before leaving the museum. If participants are comfortable, the ride home can be an enjoyable time for resting and sharing the experience with one another.

PLANNING AND EXECUTING THE POST-MUSEUM LESSON

There are several valid approaches to the post-museum lesson. In choosing the best type of lesson for a particular group one must consider learning styles, types of limitations (mental or physical), and what sort of activities seem to stimulate the group. This is an important part of the overall experience that will allow participants to take what they have learned and incorporate it into their lives.

The objectives of the post-museum visit are:

1. To give participants the opportunity to reflect verbally on the museum experience, reinforcing visual retention of objects in the exhibit

2. To use the museum exhibition as inspiration for a hands-on studio experience

Verbal Reflections

One interesting method of letting older adults with and without disabilities reflect on the field trip is the use of taped interviews. Design a series of questions that allow them to voice their feelings, opinions, and critical judgments about artwork. For example, after a trip to see an exhibit of African art, these questions could provoke interesting responses:

1. What did you enjoy most about the field trip?

2. Was this your first visit to a museum? What surprised you most about it?

3. What things did the museum do that helped you feel comfortable? What else could they have done that would have improved your experience?

4. What do you remember about the exhibit of African art?

5. Was there one piece of artwork that really impressed you? Can you describe it? Was there one that you did not like? What was displeasing about it?

6. What feeling did you experience when you looked at the African masks? Why?

7. What did you learn about African art that you did not know before the field trip?

Individual interviews can be a very rich experience for both parties. Older adults with and without disabilities often bring to art a unique viewpoint that deserves expression. If time is a factor, a group interview can be a viable option. Often participants will find it entertaining to play back the tape and listen to their own voices.

Studio Experience

Any art lesson should build on ideas participants obtained from works in the exhibition. There are many ways to be creative in designing the studio experience.

1. Use media similar to that used in the exhibit. If the field trip was to see Native American pottery, clay would be an appropriate medium for studio work. Perhaps participants can design their own ceramic vessels incorporating designs they remember seeing at the museum

2. Take an important concept from the exhibition and use it in the art lesson. For example, Impressionist painters often painted outdoors in order to capture light and shadow. Allow the group to take materials outdoors and do color sketches.

3. If the exhibition focused on one artist, find something in his or her approach to incorporate into the lesson. Romare Bearden is an artist who uses collage to re-create images of his childhood. Provide materials for the group to create their own memory collages.

4. Ask the group for ideas. Many of them may have been so inspired by what they saw that they will come up with innovative ways of interpreting it visually.

Whatever art lesson is chosen, be sure to allow time for viewing each other's work and discussing it. Perhaps there is a place at the facility for a display before individuals take their creations home or to their rooms. Many participants may want to give what they have made to family or friends as a way of sharing a special experience.

A museum field trip is a rewarding and enriching experience for each person involved. Careful planning ensures success and makes everyone want to go again and often. This is one way of getting older adults with and without disabilities out of isolated facilities and into the cultural mainstream of the community, allowing them to contribute their unique gifts of wisdom and insight.

SUMMARY

Remind the group of any special behaviors that the museum requires before leaving the facility. Go over the logistics of getting to and from the museum.

Go directly to the information desk when you arrive at the museum and let the staff know your group is there. If you have requested help, a docent should be ready and waiting to take participants directly to the exhibition area.

Help those participants who need chairs to find comfortable seating in the exhibition area.

Promote game-like activities for closer observation of artwork and for the enjoyment of participants. Speak clearly, slowly, and remember to ask questions that will encourage dialogue:

- "What is going on in this painting? How does it remind you of something you have done or felt before?"
- "How many shades of blue do you see?
- "If you could step into this painting what sort of things could you smell? Taste? Feel? Hear?"
- "Where are the people in this painting sitting?"
- "What is the largest shape in this sculpture?"

Use age-appropriate group management techniques to facilitate optimum learning.

Allow time for the group to wander freely through the gallery and make their own viewing choices.

Point out restroom facilities and allow time for a bathroom break before departure.

Alert the driver to bring the van around to the entrance of the museum.

Ask museum staff for brochures about the exhibit to give to all participants.

Suggested Readings

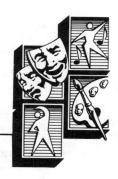

Aging

Edgerton, R.B., & Gaston, M.A. (Eds.). (1991). *I've seen it all!: Lives of older persons with mental retardation in the community.* Baltimore: Paul H. Brookes Publishing Co.

Erickson, E.H. (1980). *Identity and the life cycle.* New York: Norton.

Foster, J.M., & Gallagher, D. (1986). An exploratory study comparing depressed and nondepressed elders' coping strategies. *Journal of Gerontology, 41*(1), 91–93.

Fried, S., Van Booven, D., & MacQuarrie, C. (1993). *Older adulthood: Learning activities for understanding aging.* Baltimore: Health Professions Press.

Harper, D.C., Wadsworth, J.S., & Michael, A.L. (1987). *Elders with developmental disabilities: A working bibliography: Volume 1.* Iowa City: University of Iowa, University Affiliated Program.

Hawkins, B.A., Eklund, S.J., & Gaetani, R.P. (1989). *Aging and developmental disabilities: A training inservice package.* Bloomington: Indiana University, Institute for the Study of Developmental Disabilities.

Jacobson, J.W., & Regula, C.R. (1988). Program evaluation in community residential settings. In M.P. Janicki, M.W. Krauss, & M.M. Seltzer (Eds.), *Community residences for persons with developmental disabilities: Here to stay* (pp. 85–101). Baltimore: Paul H. Brookes Publishing Co.

Keller, M.J. (Ed.). (1991). *Activities with older adults with developmental disabilities.* Binghamton, NY: Haworth Press.

Keller, M.J., & Osgood, N.J. (Eds.). (1987). *Dynamic leisure programming with older adults.* Alexandria, VA: National Recreation and Parks Association.

Kultgen, P. (1987). *Aging and developmental disabilities.* Kansas City: University of Missouri–Kansas City, Institute for Human Development University Affiliated Program for Developmental Disabilities.

Lund, D.A. (1986). Identifying elderly with coping difficulties after two years of bereavement. *Omega Journal of Death and Dying, 16*(3), 213–224.

Malone, D.M. (1990). Aging persons with mental retardation: Identification of the needs of a special population. *Gerontology Review, 30*(3), 1–14.

McNeil, R.D., & Teague, M.L. (1987). *Aging and leisure: Vitality in later life.* Englewood Cliffs, NJ: Prentice Hall.

Moody, H.R. (1984). Reminiscence and the recovery of the public world. *Journal of Gerontological Social Work, 7*(1–2), 157–166.

Nutt, L., & Malone, D.M. (1992). Persons with lifelong disabilities in late life: Issues and approaches. In P. Wehman & P. McLaughlin (Eds.), *Handbook of developmental disabilities: A guide for best practices* (pp. 277–297). Stoneham, MA: Andover Medical Publishers.

Okun, M.A., & DiVesta, F.J. (1976). Cautiousness in adulthood as a function of age and instructions. *Journal of Gerontology, 31*(5), 571–576.

Ornstein, R., & Sobel, D. (1989). *Healthy pleasures.* Reading, MA: Addison-Wesley.

Osgood, N.J. (1982). *Life after work: Retirement, leisure, recreation, and the elderly.* New York: Praeger.

Osgood, N.J. (1987). Leisure programs. In G. Maddox (Ed.), *Encyclopedia of aging* (pp. 385–387). New York: Springer-Verlag.

Osgood, N.J. (1987). The midlife leisure renaissance: A developmental perspective. *Leisure Today, 58*(8), 35–39.

Osgood, N.J. (1989, February 24). Basics of wellness are not just for the young. *Mental Health AAHA Provider News, 4,* 5.

Osgood, N.J., & Howe, C.Z. (1984). Psychosocial aspects of leisure: A life cycle developmental perspective. *Society and Leisure, 7*(1), 175–195.

Snowden, J., & Brodaty, H. (1986). The life cycle. VIII: Old age. *Australian and New Zealand Journal of Family Therapy, 7*(2), 103–107.

Stein, S., Linn, M.W., & Stein, E.M. (1982). The relationship of self-help networks to physical and psychosocial functioning. *Journal of the American Geriatric Society, 30*(12), 764–768.

Stroud, M., & Sutton, E. (1988a). *Activities handbook and instructor's guide for Expanding options for older adults with developmental disabilities.* Baltimore: Paul H. Brookes Publishing Co.

Stroud, M., & Sutton, E. (1988b). *Expanding options for older adults with developmental disabilities: A practical guide to achieving community access.* Baltimore: Paul H. Brookes Publishing Co.

Suhart, D., Campbell, M., & Vesely, A.J. (Producers). (1977). *Art in action* [Film]. Athens: University of Georgia Center for Continuing Education.

Sweeney, T.J., & Myers, J.E. (1986). Early recollections: An Adlerian technique with older people. *Clinical Gerontologist, 4*(4), 3–12.

Van der Kolk, B.A. (1983). Psychotherapy of the elderly. General discussion: The idealizing transference and group psychotherapy with elderly patients. *Journal of Geriatric Psychiatry, 16*(1), 99–102.

Wehner, H., & Kultgen, P. (1987). *Aging in brief.* Kansas City: The University of Missouri–Kansas City, Institute for Human Development University Affiliated Program for Developmental Disabilities.

Williams, S.R. (1989). *Essentials in nutrition and diet therapy* (6th ed.). St. Louis: C.V. Mosby.

Wilson, H. (1983, April). *Increased challenge for the elderly.* Paper presented at the annual convention of the Rocky Mountain Psychological Association, Snowbird, UT (ERIC Document Reproduction Service No. 235 398).

Art

Anderson, F.E. (1978). *Art for all the children: A creative sourcebook for the impaired child.* Springfield, IL: Charles C Thomas.

Beck, A. (1975, April). NCAEE: The past is a good beginning. *School Arts,* pp. 42–43.

Butler, R.N. (1963). The life review: An interpretation of reminiscence in the aged. *Psychiatry, 26,* 65–76.

Clark, A.W. (1982). Personal and social resources as correlates of coping behaviour among the aged. *Psychological Reports, 51*(2), 577–578.

Clements, C. (1980). The rural elderly and the arts. In D.H. Hoffman, P. Greenberg, & D. Fitzner (Eds.), *Lifelong learning and the visual arts* (pp. 62–66). Reston, VA: National Art Education Association.

Clements, C., & Barret, D. (1993, April). The quality of life program: Fostering creativity in seniors through a museum experience. *Journal of Physical Education, Recreation and Dance,* pp. 48–51.

Clements, C.B., & Clements, R.D. (1984). *Art and mainstreaming.* Springfield, IL: Charles C Thomas.

Crosson, C. (1976). Art therapy with geriatric patients: Problems of spontaneity. *American Journal of Art Therapy, 15,* 51–56.

Dewdney, I. (1973). An art therapy program for geriatric patients. *American Journal of Art Therapy, 12*(4), 249–254.

Fling, S. (1982, April). *Creative health for elders through psychology and art: A pilot study.* Paper presented at the Southwestern Psychological Association. (ERIC Document Reproduction Service No. 234 326)

Greenberg, P. (1987). *Visual arts and older people: Developing quality programs.* Springfield, IL: Charles C Thomas.

Harlan, J.E. (1992). *A guide to setting up a creative art experience program for older adults with developmental disabilities.* Bloomington: Indiana University, Institute for the Study of Developmental Disabilities, University Affiliated Program.

Hoffman, D. (1982). *Pursuit of the arts activities with older Americans: An administrative and programmatic handbook.* Washington, DC: National Council on Aging, Inc.

Hoffman, D.H. (1975). A society of elders: Opportunities for expansion in art education. *Art Education, 28,* 20–22.

Hoffman, D.H. (1992). *Arts for older adults: An enhancement of life.* Englewood Cliffs, NJ: Prentice Hall.

Hoffman, D.H., Greenberg, P., & Fitzner, D. (1980). *Lifelong learning in the visual arts.* Reston, VA: National Art Education Association.

Jones, J.E. (1978). Art and elderly: An annotated biography of research and programming. *Art Education, 31*(7), 23–26, 29.

Jones, J.E. (1980a). The elderly art student: Research and the participants speak. *Art Education, 33*(7), pp. 16–19.

Jones, J.E. (1980b). On teaching art to the elderly: Research and practice. *Educational Gerontology, 5*(1), 17–31.

Katz, F.L., & Katz, E. (1978). *Creative art of the developmentally disabled.* Oakland, CA: Creative Growth.

Katz, F.L., & Katz, E. (1987). *Freedom to create.* Richmond, CA: National Institute of Arts and Disabilities.

Kauppinen, H. (1989). Discussing art with older adults. *Art Education, 42*(6), 14–19.

Lindsay, Z. (1972). *Art and the handicapped child.* New York: VanNostrand Reinhold.

Lowe, M.E. (1984). Smoke gets in your eyes, sometimes. *The Arts in Psychotherapy, 11,* 267–277.

Ludins-Katz, F., & Katz, E. (1990a). *Art & disabilities* (rev.ed.). Cambridge, MA: Brookline Books.

Ludins-Katz, F., & Katz, E. (1990b). *The creative spirit.* Richmond, CA: National Institute of Art and Disabilities.

Ludins-Katz, F., & Katz, E. (1991). *Freedom to create: Philosophy and practical experiences enabling teachers to stimulate creativity in the visual arts for disabled and nondisabled students.* Richmond, CA: National Institute of Art and Disabilities.

MacAuley, D. (1977). *Castles.* Boston: Houghton Mifflin.

Nadeau, R. (1984). Using the visual arts to expand personal creativity. In B. Warren (Ed.), *Using the creative arts in therapy* (pp. 61–80). Cambridge, MA: Brookline Books.

Potato print cards. (1987, November/December). *Programming Trends in Therapeutic Recreation, 8*(6), 26.

Robbins, A. (1987). *The artist as therapist.* New York: Human Sciences Press.

Tilley, P. (1975). *Art in the education of the subnormal child.* London: Pitman.

Creativity

Balkema, J.B. (1986). *The creative spirit: An annotated bibliography on the arts, humanities and aging.* Washington, DC: National Council on Aging.

Barsky, M. (1985). The creative powers within us. In N. Weisbery & R. Wilder (Eds.), *Creative arts with older adults* (pp. 145–154). New York: Human Sciences Press.

Blakeslee, S. (1989, March). The return of the mind: For a fit brain—learning, creativity, passion. *American Health,* pp. 94–96.

Blatner, A., & Blatner, A. (1988). *The art of play.* New York: Human Sciences Press.

Bloom, B.S. (Ed.). (1956). *Taxonomy of educational objectives: Handbook I. Cognitive domain.* New York: David McKay.

Davis, G.A. (1986). *Creativity is forever.* Dubuque, IA: Kendall/Hunt.

Dawson, A.M., & Baller, W.R. (1972). Relationship between creative activity and the health of elderly persons. *Journal of Psychology, 82,* 49–58.

de Bono, E. (1974). *Thing course for junior.* Dorset, United Kingdom: Direct Education Services.

Edwards, B. (1979). *Drawing on the right side of the brain.* Los Angeles: J.P. Tarcher, Inc.

Goff, K. (1992). Enhancing creative behavior in older adults. *Journal of Creative Behavior, 26,* 40–49.

Goff, K. (1993, March). Creativity and life satisfaction of older adults. *Educational Gerontology, 19,* 241–250.

Hanks, K., & Parry, J.A. (1983). *Wake up your creative genius.* Los Altos, CA: William Kaufman, Inc.

Koberg, D., & Bagnall, J. (1976). *The universal traveler.* Los Altos, CA: William Kaufman, Inc.

Langer, E.J. (1989). *Mindfulness.* New York: Addison-Wesley.

McCutcheon, P., & Wolf, C. (1985). *The resource guide to people, places and programss in arts and aging.* Washington, DC: The National Council on Aging, Inc.

Miller, R.S. (1988, December 1). Yes, there is a fountain of youth, flushed by creative expression. *The Los Angeles Times,* p. 25.

Osgood, N.J. (1987a, June). *Creative arts and wellness in the elderly.* Paper presented at the International Conference Toward the 21st Century, School of Physical Education and Recreation, University of British Columbia, Vancouver.

Osgood, N.J. (1987b, June). *Wellness through creative expression in late life.* Paper presented at the ICHPER Chapter, University of British Columbia.

Osgood, N.J., Meyer, B., & Orchowsly, S. (1990). The impact of creative dance and movement training on the life satisfaction of older adults: An exploratory study. *Journal of Applied Gerontology, 9*(3), 255–265.

Parris, D. (1986). Stimulating creativity through artistic inspiration. *Journal of Gerontological Nursing, 12*(5), 44.

Setlow, C.E. (1981, February). Older Americans and the arts: Analysis of current survey findings. *National Council on Aging, 1–3,* 79–104.

Siegel, B.S. (1986). *Love, medicine, & miracles.* New York: Harper & Row.

Smith, R., & Smoll, F. (1984). Leadership research in youth sports. In J.M. Silva & R.S. Weinberg (Eds.), *Psychological foundation of sport* (pp. 371–386). Champaign, IL: Human Kinetics.

Torrance, E.P. (1962). *Guiding creative talent.* Englewood Cliffs, NJ: Prentice-Hall.

Torrance, E.P. (1963). *Education and the creative potential.* Minneapolis: University of Minnesota Press.

Torrance, E.P. (1977a). Creativity in the older adult. *Creative Child and Adult Quarterly, 2,* 136–144.

Torrance, E.P. (1977b). Creativity and mental health. In S. Arieti & G. Chrzanowski (Eds.), *New dimensions in psychiatry: A world view* (Vol. 2, pp. 196–211). New York: John Wiley & Sons.

Torrance, E.P. (1978). Healing qualities of creative behavior. *Creative Child and Adult Quarterly, 3,* 146–158.

Torrance, E.P. (1979). *The search for satori and creativity.* Buffalo, NY: Creative Education Foundation.

Torrance, E.P. (1987). Part two: Recent trends in teaching children and adults to think creatively. In S.G. Isaksen (Ed.), *Frontiers of creativity research* (pp. 204–215). Buffalo, NY: Bearly Limited.

Torrance, E.P., Clements, C.B., & Goff, K. (1989). Mind-body learning among the elderly: Arts, fitness, incubation. *The Educational Forum, 54*(1), 123–133.

Torrance, E.P., & Myers, R.E. (1970). *Creative learning and teaching.* New York: Dodd-Mead.

Torrance, E.P., & Safter, H.T. (1990). *The incubation model of teaching: Getting beyond the aha!* Buffalo, NY: Bearly Limited.

Torrance, E.P., & Wright, J.A. (1988). Sociometric audience technique as a device for maximizing creativity in problem solving in large groups. *Creative Child and Adult Quarterly, 13*(3), 147–151.

Toseland, R., & Sykes, J. (1977). Senior citizen center participation and other correlates of life satisfaction. *The Gerontologist, 17*(3), 235–241.

Van Oech, R. (1983). *A whack on the side of the head.* Menlo Park, CA: Creative Think.

Veseley, A., & Torrance, E.P. (1978). *Art for older Americans.* Paper presented for Northeast Georgia Area Planning and Commission, Athens.

Wang, Y., Clements, C., Torrance, E.P., & Goff, K. (1990, June). Arts for elderly in Taiwan. *Health Magazine*, pp. 31–41.

Weinstein, B. (1983). *Twenty years to be more creative in your job.* New York: Simon & Schuster.

Weisberg, N., & Wilder, R. (1985). *Creative arts with older adults.* New York: Human Sciences Press.

Dance

American Dance Therapy Association. (1989). *Moving into a new decade: Dance/movement therapy in the 90's.* Columbia, MD: Author.

Beal, R.K., & Berryman-Miller, S. (Eds.). (1988). *Dance for the older adult.* Reston, VA: American Alliance for Health, Physical Education, Recreation and Dance.

Bernstein, P. (1981). *Theory and methods in dance-movement therapy.* Dubuque, IA: Kendall/Hunt.

Berryman-Miller, S. (1986). Benefits of dance in the process of aging and retirement for the older adult. *Activities, Adaptations & Aging, 91*, 43–47.

Berryman-Miller, S. (1988, May-June). Dance/movement: Effects on elderly self concept. *Journal of Physical Education, Recreation and Dance, 59*(5), 42–46.

Berryman-Miller, S., & Beal, R. (1982). *Focus on dance XI: Dance and the older adult.* Waldorf, MD: AAHPERD Publications.

Clark, B.A. (1986, October). Exercise programs for older adults: What they should know to get started. *Journal of Physical Education, Recreation, and Dance, 57*(8), 63–65.

De Guzman, J.A. (1979, April). Dance as a contributor to cardiovascular fitness and alteration of body composition. *Journal of Physical Education, Recreation, and Dance, 50*(4), 88.

Fitt, S., & Riordan, A. (1980). *Focus on dance IX: Dance for the handicapped.* Waldorf, MD: AAHPERD Publications.

Gorman, D. , & Brown, B. (1986, January). Fitness and aging: An overview. *Journal of Physical Education, Recreation, and Dance, 57*(54), 50–51.

Gustafson, G., Pfetzing, D., & Zawolrow, E. (1980). *Signing exact English.* Los Alamitos, CA: Modern Signs Press.

Hecox, B. (1983, May). Movement activities for older adults. *Journal of Physical Education, Recreation and Dance, 54*(50) 47–48.

Keller, M.J., & Turner, N.D. (1986). Creating wellness programs with older people: A process for therapeutic recreators. *Therapeutic Recreation Journal, 20*(4), 6–14.

Kratz, L.E. (1973). *Movement without sight: Physical activity and dance for the visually handicapped.* Palo Alto, CA: Peck Publications.

Lerman, L. (1984). *Teaching dance to senior adults.* Springfield, IL: Charles C Thomas.

Levy, F.J. (1992). *Dance/movement therapy: A healing art.* Reston, VA: National Dance Association.

Lidner, E.C., & Harpaz, L. (1983, May). Shared movement programs: Children and older adults. *Journal of Physical Education, Recreation and Dance, 54*(50), 49–50.

Lidner, E.C., Harpaz, L., & Samberg, S. (1979). *Therapeutic dance/movement: Expressive activities for older adults.* New York: Human Sciences Press.

Lopez, R. (1983, May). Guidelines for using dance with older adults. *Journal of Physical Education, Recreation and Dance, 54*, 44–45.

Metal-Corbin, J. (1983, May). Shared movement programs: College students and older adults. *Journal of Physical Education, Recreation and Dance, 50*(54), 46.

Osgood, N.J., Meyer, B., & Orchowsly, S. (1990). The impact of creative dance and movement training on the life satisfaction of older adults: An exploratory study. *Journal of Applied Gerontology, 9*(3), 255–265.

Payne, H. (Ed.). (1992). *Dance movement therapy: Theory and practice.* New York: Tavistock/Routledge.

Pruett, D.M. (1983, May). Dance for older adults. *Journal of Physical Education, Recreation and Dance, 54*(5), 43–51.

Siegel, E.V. (1984). *Dance-movement therapy: The mirror of our souls. A psychoanalytic approach.* New York: Human Sciences Press.

Smith, E.L., & Zook, S.K. (1986, January). The aging process: Benefits of physical activity. *Journal of Physical Education, Recreation, and Dance, 57*, 32–34.

Sneegas, J.J. (1985, October). *Components of life satisfaction in middle and later life adults: Perceived social competence, leisure participation, and leisure satisfaction.* Paper presented at the Research Symposium of the National Recreation and Park Association National Congress, Dallas.

Wethered, A. (1973). *Movement and drama in therapy: The therapeutic use of movement, drama, and music.* Boston: Plays.

Van Zandt, S., & Lorenson, L. (1985). You're not too old to dance: Creative movement and older adults. *Activities, Adaptation & Aging, 6*(4), 121–130.

Drama

Bennett, R., & Gurland, B. (1981). *The acting out elderly.* New York: Haworth Press.

Bright, R. (1981). *Practical planning in music therapy for the aged.* New York: Musicgraphics.

Burger, I. (1980). *Creative drama for senior adults.* Wilton, CT: Morehouse Barlow.

Butler, R.N. (1968). The life review: An interpretation of reminiscence in the aged. In B.L. Neugarten (Ed.), *Middle age and aging.* Chicago: University of Chicago Press.

Clark, P., & Osgood, N.J. (1985). *Seniors on stage: The impact of applied theatre techniques on the elderly.* New York: Praeger Special Studies.

Cornish, R. (1981). *Senior adult theatre: The American Theatre Association handbook.* University Park: Pennsylvania State University Press.

Cranston, J. (1975). *Dramatic imagination.* Eureka, CA: Interface California Corp.

Davis, B.W. (1985, June). The impact of creative drama training on psychological states of older adults: An exploratory study. *The Gerontologist, 25*(3), 315–321.

Davis, B.W. (1987). Some roots and relatives of creative drama as an enrichment activity for older adults. *Educational Gerontology, 4*(13), 297–306.

Douglas, D. (1981). *Accent on rhythm: Music activities for the aged.* Salem, OR: La Roux Enterprises.

Fine, B. (1987, January/February). Saving family memories on cassette tapes. *Programming Trends in Therapeutic Recreation, 8*(1), 6–7.

Goodwin, D.A. (1985). An investigation into the efficacy of creative drama as a method for teaching social skills to mentally retarded youth and adults. *Children's Theater Review, 2*(34), 23–26.

Gray, P.G. (1974). *Dramatics for the elderly: A guide for residential care settings and senior centers.* New York: Teachers College Press.

Harbin, S. (1976). *Dramatic activities for the elderly.* Ann Arbor: University of Michigan/Wayne State University, Institute of Gerontology.

Harmon, B. (1981). *How to get a drama group off the ground and out on the town.* Available from Health and Aging Services, Inc., 775 Main Street, Suite 221, Buffalo, NY 14203.

Huston, N.B. (1968). *Stage.* Available from Educational Service, Inc., P.O. Box 219, Stevensville, MI 49127.

Kaminsky, M. (1984). The uses of reminiscence: A discussion of the formative literature. *Journal of Gerontological Social Work, 7*(1–2), 137–156.

Koch, K. (1977). *Never told anybody: Teaching poetry writing in a nursing home.* New York: Random House.

Kubie, S., & Landeau, G. (1969). *Group work with the aged.* New York: International University Press.

Mayer-Bliebery, S. (1987, May/June). Lift our spirits. *Programming Trends in Therapeutic Recreation, 8*(3), 3–4.

M'buzi, M. (1986). *Red clay and restructured wood.* Atlanta: Expansion Press.

Monaghan, T.A. (1976). *Releasing playfulness in adults through creative drama.* Ann Arbor, MI: University Microfilms.

Osgood, N.J. (1985). *Seniors on stage: The impact of applied theatre techniques on the elderly.* New York: Praeger.

Osgood, N.J. (1988). Impact of creative dramatics on the life satisfaction of elderly blacks. *Journal of Minority Aging, 9*(1), 60–71.

Pearlman, W.D. (1990). Psychodrama: Discovering new meaning in personal drama. *New Directions in Adult and Continuing Education, 45,* 27–36.

Pemberton-Billing, R.N., & Clegg, J.D. (1968). *Teaching drama.* London: University of London Press.

Planning for the holiday scene. (1987, November/December). *Programming Trends in Therapeutic Recreation, 8*(6), 26.

Producing inexpensive special events for senior citizens. (1989, January/February). *Programming Trends in Therapeutic Recreation, 1,* 7–12.

Progressive games carnival. (1987, July/August). *Programming Trends in Therapeutic Recreation, 8*(4), 16–23.

Salter, V. (1987, November/December). Bean bag activities. *Programming Trends in Therapeutic Recreation, 8*(6), 30.

Self, D. (1976). *A practical guide to drama in the secondary school.* London: Wardlock Educational.

Shaftel, F.R., & Shaftel, G. (1967). *Roleplaying for social values: Decision-making in the social studies.* Englewood Cliffs, NJ: Prentice Hall.

Shaw, A.M., & Perks, W. (Eds.). (1981). *Perspectives: A handbook in drama and theater by, with and for handicapped individuals.* Washington, DC: American Theater Association.

Stewig, J.W. (1973). *Spontaneous drama: A language art.* Columbus, OH: Charles E. Merrill.

Swink, D. F. (1985). Psychodramatic treatment for deaf people. *American Annals for the Deaf, 4*(13), 272–277.

Thurman, A.H., & Piggins, C.A. (1982). *Drama activities with older adults: A handbook for leaders.* New York: Haworth Press.

Trivial pursuits. (1987, January/February). *Programming Trends in Therapeutic Recreation, 8*(1), 33–34.

The twelve days of Christmas ornaments. (1987, November/December). *Programming Trends in Therapeutic Recreation, 8*(6), 5.

Vorenberg, B.L. (1987). *New plays for mature actors: An anthology.* Morton Grove, IL: Coach House Press.

Fitness

Bogdonoff, M.D. (1983). *Forever fit: The exercise program for staying young.* Boston: Little, Brown.

Corbin, D.E., & Metal-Corbin, J. (1983). *Reach for it: A handbook of exercise and dance activities for older adults.* Dubuque, IA: Eddie Bowers Publishing Co.

Crawford, M.E. (1987). *Therapeutic recreation and adapted physical activities for mentally retarded individuals.* Englewood Cliffs, NJ: Prentice Hall.

Flatten, K., Wilhite, B., & Reyes-Watson, E. (1988). *Exercise activities for the elderly.* New York: Springer.

Frankel, L.J., & Richard, B.B. (1980). *Be alive as long as you live.* New York: Lippincott & Crowell.

Garnet, E.D. (1982). *Chair exercise manual.* Princeton, NJ: Princeton Book Co.

Greninger, L.O., & Kinney, M.B. (1988). *Therapeutic exercises for older adults.* Dubuque, IA: Eddie Bowers Publishing Co.

Gueldner, S.H., & Spradley, J. (1989). Outdoor walking lowers fatigue. *Journal of Gerontological Nursing, 14*(10), 6–12.

Hoeger, W.K., & Hoeger, S.A. (1992). *Lifetime physical fitness and wellness.* Englewood, CO: Morton Publishing Co.

Hurley, O. (1988). *Safe therapeutic exercise for the frail elderly.* Albany, NY: The Center for the Study of Aging.

IOX Assessment Associates. (1988). *Program evaluation handbook: Physical fitness promotion.* Los Angeles: Center for Health Promotion and Education, and the Office of Disease Prevention and Health Promotion.

Jacobson, E. (1956). *Progressive relaxation.* Chicago: University of Chicago Press.

Knopf, K.G., & Downs, S.B. (1989). *Fitness over fifty.* Dubuque, IA: Kendall/Hunt.

LaLanne, E., & Benyo, R. (1989). *Fitness after 50 workout.* New York: Stephen Breene Press, Pelham Books.

Lasko, P., & Knopf, K. (1988). *Adapted exercises for the disabled adult.* Dubuque, IA: Eddie Bowers Publishing Co.

Olsson, R.H., Jr. (1987, May/June). The relaxation effect: An automated program for measuring and controlling stress. *Programming Trends in Therapeutic Recreation, 8*(3), 26–28.

Piscopo, J. (1985). *Fitness and aging.* New York: Macmillan.

Rikkers, R. (1986). *Seniors on the move.* Champaign, IL: Human Kinetics Publishers.

Strem, L. (1989, March/April). Take a walk. *Programming Trends in Therapeutic Recreation, 10*(2), 3–4.

Williams, M.H. (1990). *Lifetime fitness and wellness: A personal choice.* Dubuque, IA: William C. Brown.

Woodard, B. (1989, July/August). Fitness for seniors. *Programming Trends in Therapeutic Recreation, 10*(4), 8–11.

Program Planning

Adler, A. (1958). *The education of the individual.* New York: Philosophical Library.

Coleman, D., & Salter, V. (1989, January/February). Leisure education. *Programming Trends in Therapeutic Recreation, 10*(1), 13–16.

Cotten, P.D., Casey, J., Jr., Ezell, D.S., & Gardner, M. (1990a). *Pre-retirement training curriculum: Guide and pictorial guide.* Sanatorium, MS: Boswell Mental Retardation Center.

Cotten, P.D., Casey, J., Jr., Ezell, D.S., & Gardner, M. (1990b). *Pre-retirement training student handbook.* Sanatorium, MS: Boswell Mental Retardation Center.

Dattilo, J. (1991). *Leisure education program planning: A systematic approach.* State College, PA: Venture Publishing.

Dattilo, J., & Murphy, W.D. (1987). *Behavior modification in therapeutic recreation: An introductory learning manual.* State College, PA: Venture Publishing.

Duke, G. (1989, March/April). Planning recreational activities for the elderly in long term facilities. *Programming Trends in Therapeutic Recreation, 10*(2), 27–29.

Flatten, K., Wilhite, B., & Reyes-Watson, E. (1988). *Recreation activities for the elderly.* New York: Springer-Verlag.

Greenblatt, F.S. (1988). *Therapeutic recreation for the long term care facilities.* New York: Human Sciences Press.

Hastings, L.E. (1981). *Complete handbook of activities and recreational programs for nursing homes.* Englewood Cliffs, NJ: Prentice Hall.

Jones, L. (1987). *Activities for the older mentally retarded/developmentally disabled.* Akron, OH: Exploration Series Press.

LePore, P., & Janicki, M.P. (1990). *The wit to win: How to integrate older persons with developmental disabilities into community aging programs.* Albany: New York State Office for the Aging.

Merrill, T. (1971). *Activities for the aged and infirm: A handbook for the untrained worker.* Springfield, IL: Charles C Thomas.

Pierce, N., & Burgio, M. (1981). *Evaluation of the liberal arts program of the international study of older adults.* (ERIC Document Reproduction Service No. 210 056)

Program planning based on resident needs. (1989, March/April). *Programming Trends in Therapeutic Recreation, 10*(2), 16–18.

Salter, V. (1987, September/October). Warmer uppers or get to know your neighbor. *Programming Trends in Therapeutic Receation, 8*(5), 10–12.

Sanchez, B. (1987, July/August). Back to life: Rediscovering the value of receation and leisure. *Programming Trends in Therapeutic Recreation, 8*(4), 3–4.

Stumbo, N.J., & Thompson, S.R. *Leisure education: A manual of activities and resources.* State College, PA: Venture Publishing.

Torrance, E.P., & Safter, H.T. (1990). *The incubation model of teaching: Getting beyond the aha!* Buffalo, NY: Bearly Limited.

Yarbourgh, E.S. (1987, March/April). A new way to reach the unreached families of long term care residents. *Programming Trends in Therapeutic Recreation, 8*(2), 3–6.

Zgola, J.M. (1987). *Doing things: A guide to programming activities for persons with Alzheimer's disease and related disorders.* Baltimore: Johns Hopkins University Press.

Index

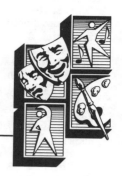